CH

D0442751

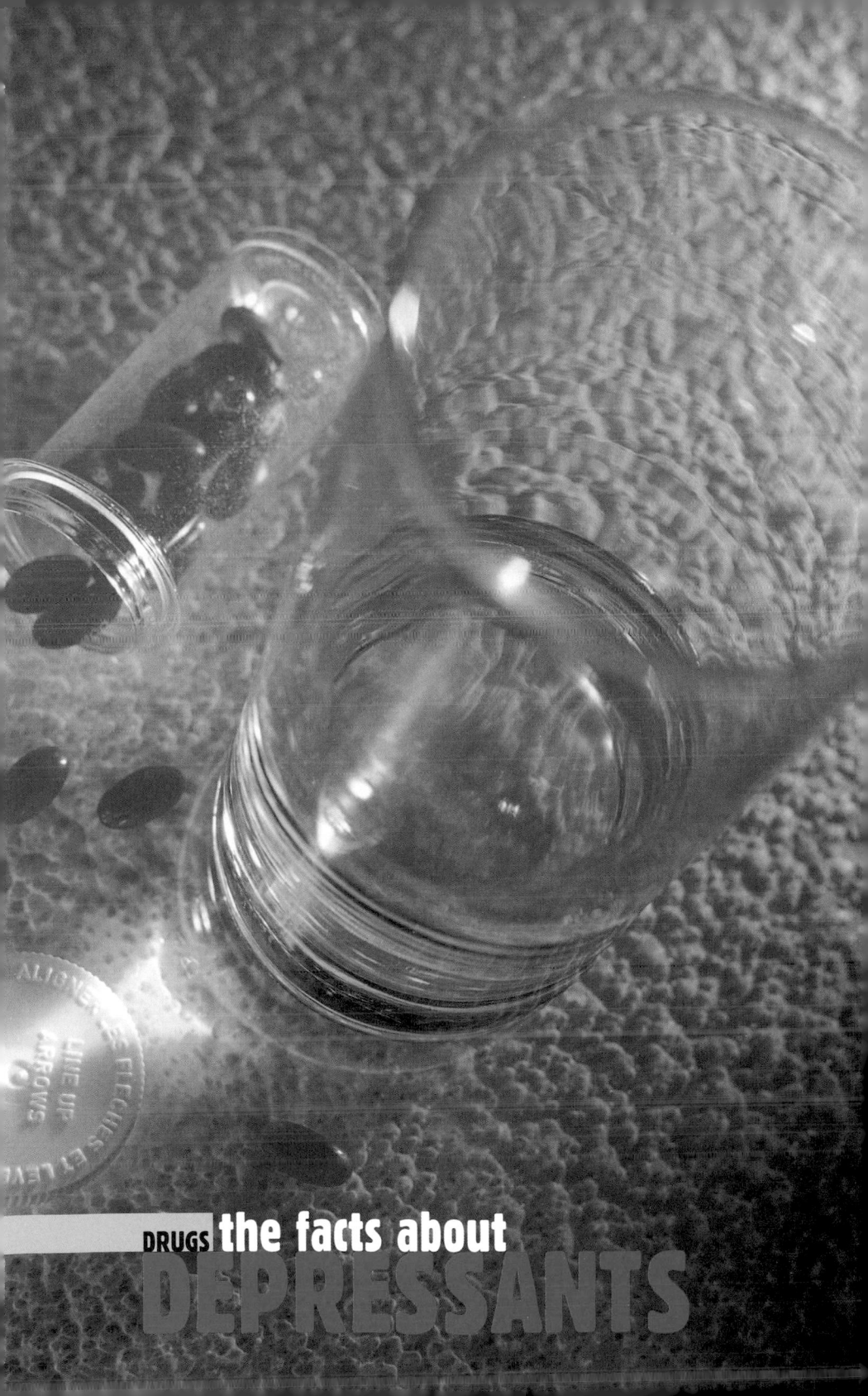

DRUGS the facts about
DEPRESSANTS

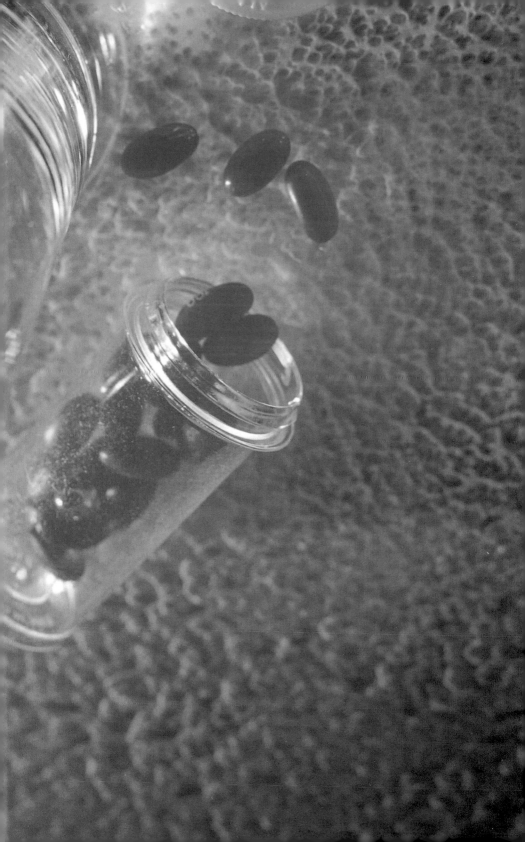

DRUGS **the facts about**
DEPRESSANTS

LORRIE KLOSTERMAN

Marshall Cavendish
Benchmark
New York

This book is dedicated especially to young people, who are growing up with thousands of medicines and drugs around and lots of conflicting advice about what is good and what is bad. May
you continue educating yourselves so you can make informed decisions, stay safe, and become
who you most want to be.

Series Consultant: Dr. Amy Kohn, Chief Executive Officer, YWCA of White Plains and Central
Westchester, New York.
Thanks to John M. Roll, Ph.D., Director of Behavioral Pharmacology at UCLA Integrated
Substance Abuse Programs, for his expert reading of this manuscript.

Marshall Cavendish Benchmark
99 White Plains Road
Tarrytown, NY 10591
www.marshallcavendish.us
Text copyright © 2006 by Marshall Cavendish Corporation
Illustrations copyright © 2006 by Marshall Cavendish Corporation
Library of Congress Cataloging-in-Publication Data
Klosterman, Lorrie.
The facts about depressants / by Lorrie Klosterman.
p. cm. — (Drugs)
Summary: "Describes the history, characteristics, legal status, and abuse
of the tranquilizers and downers (depressants)"—Provided by publisher.
Includes bibliographical references and index.
ISBN 0-7614-1976-4
1. Tranquilizing drugs. I. Title. II. Series: Drugs (Benchmark Books)
RM333.K56 2005
615'.7882—dc22
2005001729
Photo research by Joan Meisel

Cover photo: Royalty-Free/Corbis

Alamy: Phototake, 34; Mark Baigent, 55; Tina Manley, 56; Chris Gibson, 72. Corbis: Royalty-
Free, 1, 2-3, 5; Roy Morsch, 6; Reuters, 13; Bettmann, 45; Shepard Sherbell, 59. Getty Images:
Sandro Miller/Taxi, 25; Digital Vision, 26; Time Life Pictures, 40; Hulton Archive, 43. Photo
Researchers, Inc.: David Gifford, 28; Ray Simons, 32; Ed Young, 37.
Printed in China
1 3 5 6 4 2

CONTENTS

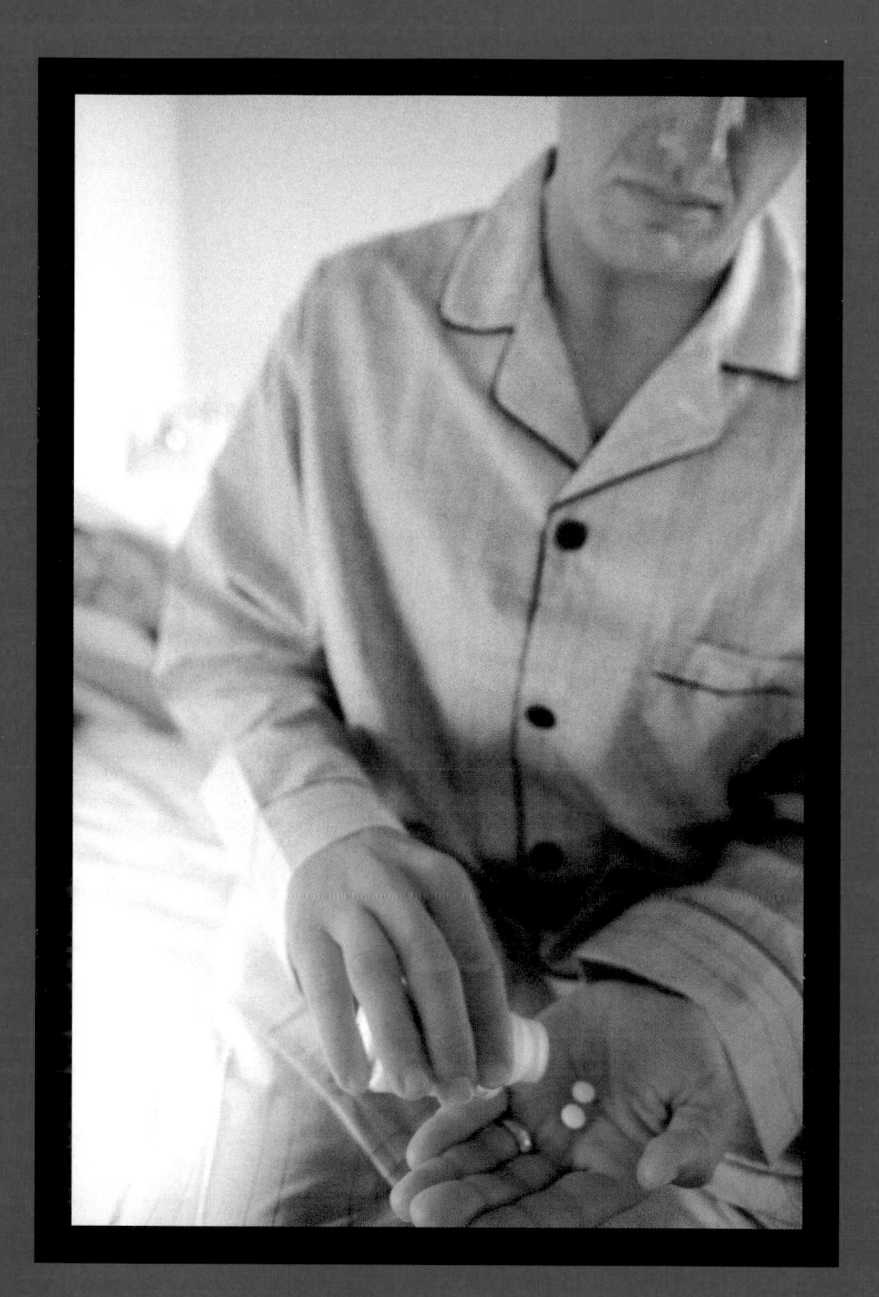

DEPRESSANTS ARE OFTEN PRESCRIBED FOR PEOPLE WHO SUFFER FROM INSOMNIA.

WHAT ARE DEPRESSANTS?

THE PURPOSE OF this book is to introduce the reader to the world of depressants, both as medical tools and as drugs of abuse. In the medical world, they have many names: sedatives, hypnotics, soporifics, tranquilizers, anesthetics, antianxiety medications, and anxiolytics. In the illegal drug trade depressants are often called downers, along with dozens of other nicknames for each particular drug.

A "depressant" doesn't sound like something anybody would want to take, because the name suggests it might make a person depressed or unhappy. But these drugs are named for a different meaning of the word *depress*, which is to slow down or diminish something—in this case, the activities of the brain and spinal cord. The brain and spinal cord together are known as the central nervous system, or CNS. The CNS controls virtually everything that keeps a person alive. Not only does it automatically control such things as breathing, blood flow, and digestion, it also makes a person's life unique and rich with emotions, thoughts, memories, speech, artistic expression, and so much more. All of those things take place in the CNS, and especially in the brain.

The drugs discussed in this book are CNS depressants. They include some very common medicines that are helping many people deal with health problems or emotional difficulties. Others are an important part of the mixture of medicines used during surgical procedures.

Depressants have been available for a little over a hundred years. Old movies featured distressed people fumbling for a bottle of pills in the bedside drawer, then popping some in their mouth and settling in for a night's sleep. Today, depressants come mostly as pills, but also as liquids and powders, and are popular medicines to relieve anxiety, sleeplessness, and more.

One of the most common reasons people take depressant drugs is insomnia—difficulty falling asleep or staying asleep. Another is anxiety—feelings of worry, agitation, or fear that are strong enough to prevent leading a normal life.

Antidepressants

It is important to point out that depressants are very different drugs than antidepressants. Antidepressants, also in common use today, are medicines that help a person overcome depression—a serious emotional and psychological state of deep despair. Depressants and antidepressants work differently in the brain, and have very different influences on a person's mood. For some depressed people, however, depressants can establish a feeling of calm that can help with some aspects of their emotional turmoil.

It is common for a person to suffer from both insomnia and anxiety. Sometimes the causes of these problems are obvious and temporary, and depressants are valuable tools in helping a person get past a rough period in life while steps are taken to eliminate those causes. Other times the causes aren't clear. And although taking depressants relieves the sleeplessness or the anxiety, they don't fix the underlying problems. In fact, taking drugs can become a way of avoiding problems and prolonging them.

Many of the effects that depressants have on the brain are related to each other, and only differ in degree. For example, some mild depressants can relax someone who had been feeling anxious or hyperactive. Others cause a sense of being "foggy" and slow. Yet other depressants cause sleepiness and muscle weakness, to the degree that a person is unable to control movements and speech. Stronger depressants cause deep sleep or unconsciousness. Depressants in overdose can lead to coma and even death.

Some depressant drugs have more than one kind of effect. For example, a sedative is a depressant that calms nervousness. But it might also make a person quite sleepy. Or a sleeping pill, meant to make a person fall asleep quickly and to sleep soundly, can also interfere with muscle control, causing clumsiness and weakness. Depressants can have more than one effect on a person for several reasons. One is the chemical nature of the drug itself. Another is that different people can react differently to the same drug. The physical health or emotional condition of a person can influence a drug's effects. Other medications or substances taken at the same time can also influence how a depressant will affect someone.

Why People Take Depressants

Even though a single depressant drug can have more than one effect on a person, it can be useful to talk about each kind of effect separately. And researchers who are creating new depressant drugs are attempting to find chemicals that have one effect only. That way, a patient can be given just the right medicine to help them,

MEDICAL TERMS FOR DEPRESSANT DRUGS

CNS Depressant	Tranquilizer
Sedative	Anesthetic
Hypnotic	Antianxiety medication
Sleeping Pill	Anxiolytic
Soporific	

without causing changes in other things that don't need fixing.

Sedatives

Sedatives are depressants that are intended to make a person feel calm and relaxed when something upsetting has happened. They are not meant to be taken for a long time, or to help with problems like anxiety attacks or insomnia. Sedatives may cause sleepiness, but that is not their main intent. The most common reason for taking a sedative is to ease an overwhelming sense of worry, fear, sadness, or other emotion that is getting in the way of daily life.

Virtually everyone at some point in life feels powerful, troubling emotions. That doesn't mean everyone needs a sedative. But sometimes a person feels so overwhelmed with strong feelings that a doctor's assistance with medication seems

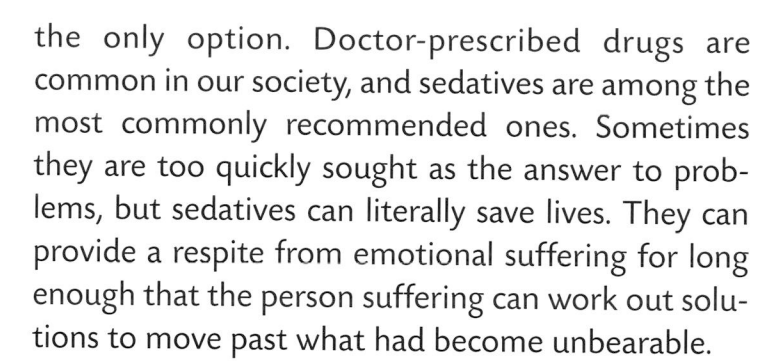

the only option. Doctor-prescribed drugs are common in our society, and sedatives are among the most commonly recommended ones. Sometimes they are too quickly sought as the answer to problems, but sedatives can literally save lives. They can provide a respite from emotional suffering for long enough that the person suffering can work out solutions to move past what had become unbearable.

Antianxiety Medicines

Another reason a person might take a depressant drug is to combat anxiety. This abnormally intense sense of fear often causes physical symptoms like sweating and an increased pulse rate. It may sound odd to turn to drugs in these instances, because such feelings are a common life experience. But antianxiety medications, or anxiolytics, are not prescribed for everyday nervousness. For instance, a student who must present a report in front of the class may feel anxious, with cold and sweaty hands, uncontrollable trembling, dry mouth, stomach upset, and so on. But that isn't something needing drugs. Very different is the constant or recurring feeling of overwhelming anxiety that some people experience—a gnawing nervousness, panic, dread, or even fear for their lives, which occurs under circumstances that don't seem to warrant such intense reactions, or for no apparent reason at all.

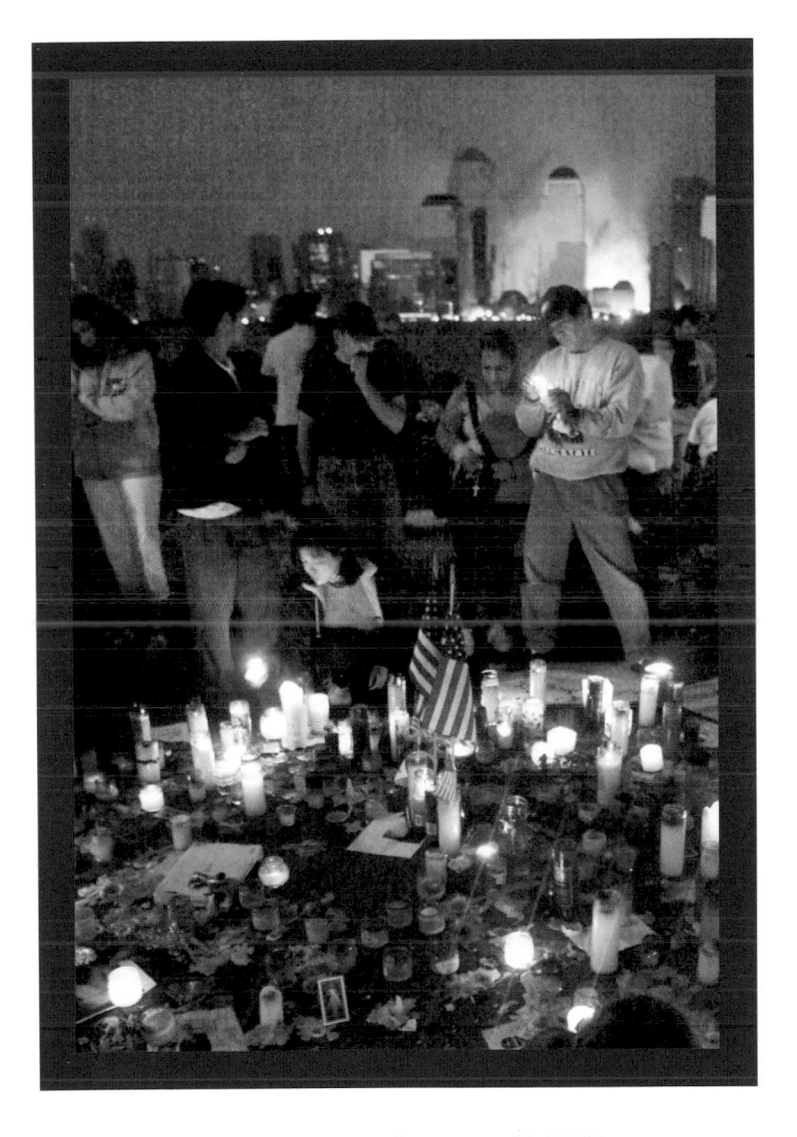

AFTER THE TERRORIST ATTACKS ON SEPTEMBER 11, 2001, MANY PEOPLE SUFFERED FROM INCREASED ANXIETY. DEPRESSANTS CAN BE EFFECTIVE IN TREATING A NUMBER OF ANXIETY DISORDERS.

Depressants used to treat anxiety disorders

GENERIC NAME	BRAND NAME
Alprazolam	Xanax
Buspirone	Buspar
Chlordiazepoxide	Librium
Clonazepam	Klonopin
Diazepam	Valium
Halazepam	Paxipam
Lorazepam	Ativan
Oxazepam	Serax
Prazepam	Centrax
Quazepam	Doral

When these feelings are serious enough or frequent enough to interfere with a person's life, it is considered to be a medical condition called anxiety disorder. There are different kinds of anxiety disorders, and about 19 million people in the United States have one of them or a combination of them. Anxiety disorders include phobias, post-traumatic stress disorder, panic attacks, and obsessive-compulsive disorder. In addition, a person may have a generalized anxiety disorder, an inexplicable, haunting sense of dread that something bad is going to happen.

Anxiety disorders can result from an inborn imbalance in brain chemicals and tend to run in families. But they also can develop after an intensely disturbing event. For example, someone who has been the victim of a violent crime may become fearful of going out alone or of doing anything that is similar to the situation in which the crime occurred. This would be an example of post-traumatic stress disorder. Soldiers who have been in active combat in a war can suffer from this form of anxiety disorder, as can people who live in a war-torn country.

Sometimes a person's anxiety isn't about a past event but a specific thing or circumstance that is ongoing. This condition is called a phobia. Often the word *phobia* is attached to another word to describe the specific fear, such as arachnophobia (*arachno*—refers to "spider"). That particular phobia isn't very important in most people's lives, and just causes a little chill now and then. But something like agoraphobia, the fear of being outside and in public places, can actually cause people to lock themselves in the house and come out only in dire need. Such people will arrange to have all their food and supplies

Tranquilizers

The term *tranquilizer* sometimes is used to refer to an antianxiety medicine. The term *minor tranquilizer* means a drug with a mild effect on the CNS, whereas a *major tranquilizer* means one with a strong depressant effect. Those terms aren't used much anymore, but it remains true that some depressants are milder, merely making a person feel calm, while others can induce sleep, cause muscle relaxation, or even unconsciousness.

delivered to the house, for example. This may sound like the person is just being antisocial, but very intense and serious physical reactions—like a racing heartbeat, inability to breathe properly, feeling faint, and trembling—may result if the person is forced outside against their will, or even imagines that idea. People who have serious phobias improve with the aid of a depressant drug that lowers the intensity of their fear. This helps them function in society well enough to learn other, long-lasting ways to deal with their fears.

Another kind of anxiety disorder is a panic attack (also called anxiety attack, or panic disorder). This is different than other anxiety problems in that it happens very suddenly. It is an overwhelming sense of fear that can cause physical symptoms that are so serious that they often are confused with a heart attack. They include irregular heartbeat, chest pain, dizziness, shortness of breath, nausea, numbness, tingling, as well as a feeling of "going crazy" and of dying. For many people with agoraphobia, an underlying problem is that they have a history of panic attacks, and they fear they will have an attack while away from home, where they can't take care of themselves properly or get the right kind of help.

Panic attacks are about twice as common in women as men and usually appear for the first time when a person is a young adult. About half of all people who develop panic attacks have the first one before the age of twenty-four. They usually happen repeatedly over a person's life and can occur several times a week. In addition to the agony of the panic episodes themselves, people with panic attacks often are worried between episodes, always wondering when another might suddenly happen. That can lead to an avoidance of places or social events that have triggered attacks in the past, and lead to agoraphobia.

Depressant drugs can help people with any of these forms of anxiety disorder, but they aren't prescribed as often as they used to be. Instead, doctors have found that other drugs (certain kinds of antidepressants) are very effective, and they can be taken for months or years to combat anxiety symptoms. Still, the depressant drugs continue to be helpful with sudden anxiety symptoms because they act very quickly to calm a per-

The Healing Power of Proper Depressant Use

Tamara first stared having panic attacks at age nine-teen—a typical age for anxiety disorders to appear. She was initially prescribed depressants to help her cope. "I felt like I was trying to move through Jello," she says. "I could only function on the very simplest of levels. There was no intellectual activity. Everything was slow, and it felt like it took so much effort to take steps." She stopped taking it. "I felt so horrible while taking it that I didn't take another kind of antianxiety drug for years."

But then, years later, she had a nervous breakdown—panic attacks that would not stop. Instead of the hour-long episodes she used to have, her anxiety was constant. "On a scale of 1 to 10, I was on an 11 all the time," she recalls. "My nerves were fried from being in that panic state all the time. I was also having severe acid reflux because of my nervous condition, and throwing up, which made me even more nervous." Her anxiety got to the point where she couldn't leave the house. She had to quit her job. Her doctor prescribed another medication along with an antidepressant drug. The doctor also insisted she start working with a therapist to work on the emotional stress behind her condition.

"My intellect was working just fine, my senses were working fine, but it made my body very relaxed." It suited her need to stay clearheaded and quick thinking. She would take one in the morning and just lay in bed while it took effect. She didn't take it for long, but it helped her get back on her feet. Unfortunately, Tamara's panic attacks have been returning, but the therapy helps her deal with them. A doctor has suggested drugs again, and she has a prescription on hand, just in case. "It's very much like a security blanket. I know I have a recipe for comfort in the event of a really serious panic attack."

For Tamara, taking the drug was never a lifestyle change. She never had any addictive feelings or withdrawal problems, though she knows people who have. It's helped her to stay functioning while doing the therapeutic work to help heal the underlying emotional causes. She now has a very healthy perspective about her condition.

"The anxiety has created so much humiliation in my life, but it has become a valuable tool. If I'm having attacks now, it means I'm not doing as good a job as I could to take care of myself. I know that the panic attacks are a volcano of emotion. They are telling me there's something that needs paying attention to."

son down. Anyone who is taking a drug for an anxiety disorder should also work with a mental health professional (therapist, psychologist, or psychiatrist) to discover the underlying causes of their anxiety.

Some antianxiety medicines can help prevent seizures in people with epilepsy, which is a brain disorder that causes episodes of muscle contractions all over the body that can be intense enough to cause injury.

Sleeping Aids

Depressants that cause sleepiness are known as sleeping pills, hypnotics, and, less often, soporifics. They are recommended by a doctor for someone who is having trouble falling asleep or staying asleep on their own. And while there may be many things a person could do besides taking a drug to sleep better, some patients seek a quick fix and are able to find doctors who will suggest medication right away. Increasingly, however, problems such as dependence and side effects are making consumers more cautious of even getting started on sleeping pills.

There are many reasons a person might have trouble sleeping. Being in physical pain is one. When something is hurting, it can be impossible to sleep well, even though sleep is just what a body needs to heal. Getting good, solid sleep can speed the healing process and recovery time for an injury or illness.

Depressants commonly used to treat insomnia

There may be more than one medication on the market that contain a specific drug. Listed here are just some examples.

GENERIC NAME	BRAND NAME
Estazolam	ProSom
Flurazepam	Dalmane
Quazepam	Doral
Temazepam	Restoril
Triazolam	Halcion
Zaleplon	Sonata
Zolpidem	Ambien
Hydroxyzine	Atarax; Vistaril

A specific event that has a devastating emotional impact is another common reason a person can't sleep. It could be something very sad, like the death of a loved one, or something extremely worrisome, like the sudden loss of a job. In circumstances like these, it can be difficult to stop the whirlwind of painful thoughts and feelings long enough to allow the brain to shut down into sleep mode.

Another reason some people have trouble falling asleep easily is because they lead such busy, stressful lives that they can't settle down at night. Many people are attempting to do more and more each day in an effort to keep up with paying bills, caring for family, maintaining a residence and possessions, getting exercise, and a whole list of other "shoulds." For some, the need is real. Without working two jobs, for example, some single parents don't have enough money to pay all the bills. For other people, though, the stressful and frantic nature of their lifestyle is something they might be able to change. If a person's lifestyle is so troubling that it takes drugs to fall asleep, then maybe the lifestyle needs to be altered, not the brain's chemistry.

Sleeping aids are not meant to be taken on a regular basis. They are supposed to help a person get proper sleep through a rough period, maybe for as long as a week or two. During that time, it is hoped that whatever is preventing a normal ability to sleep will be resolved. Exceptions to this are people with certain mental disorders for which doctors and psychiatrists feel a chemical is required to help the CNS carry out its pattern of wakefulness and sleep. Also, people who are taking medications or illegal drugs that are stimulants—substances that do the opposite of depressants—may be too hyperactive and agitated from the stimulant to sleep and will take a sleeping aid to counteract the artificial "high" created by the stimulant.

People who need help sleeping may also feel they need a sedative or antianxiety drug during the day. Indeed, there are tragedies in life that can be so difficult to bear, for a time, that medication both day and night is valuable help. It is a blessing that drugs exist to help people in this way. At the same time, patients can become so accustomed to taking depressants to remain calm or to sleep that they don't believe they can manage without them. What's more, people who stop taking depressants have a very serious withdrawal reaction, which can include feeling extremely agitated and troubled— even more than before they took the drugs.

Medical Procedures and Surgery

Depressant drugs have many uses in the medical world. A depressant may be offered to a person before getting teeth pulled or having a minor surgical procedure, to reduce any anxiousness about the procedure. (Dentists have the authority to use and prescribe depressant drugs, just as doctors do.) People who are going to have major surgery, where they are made unconscious by drugs known as general anesthetics, usually are given depressants beforehand to help them relax. Some depressants can be used at high doses as general anesthetics themselves. Depressants are also given to most patients who are in a hospital's intensive care unit, which is where people with very serious illnesses or injuries are cared for and patients recover just after surgery.

The ability of some depressants to relax muscles is helpful for medical testing and for surgery. For example, depressants help patients, especially children, to remain still during medical procedures that are painless but a little scary, or that may take a while, such as getting an MRI (magnetic resonance imaging) scan, which provides pictures of internal organs like the brain, chest, or abdomen. Depressants are also added to the mix of drugs given to a person undergoing surgery, to prevent muscular reflexes, like jerking an arm or tensing muscles, which sometimes happens even though the person is unconscious.

How Do People Obtain Depressants?

Almost all depressants must be obtained by prescription, meaning that a doctor must recommend, or prescribe, the drug to a patient. The doctor will write a note giving that person permission to buy the drug. The patient then goes to a pharmacist, shows the doctor's note, and is allowed to purchase the drug.

The purchase of depressants is controlled this way because people easily become dependent on them, meaning that they need to continue taking the drug because the body will go through intense physical reaction (withdrawal) without it, or because of strong

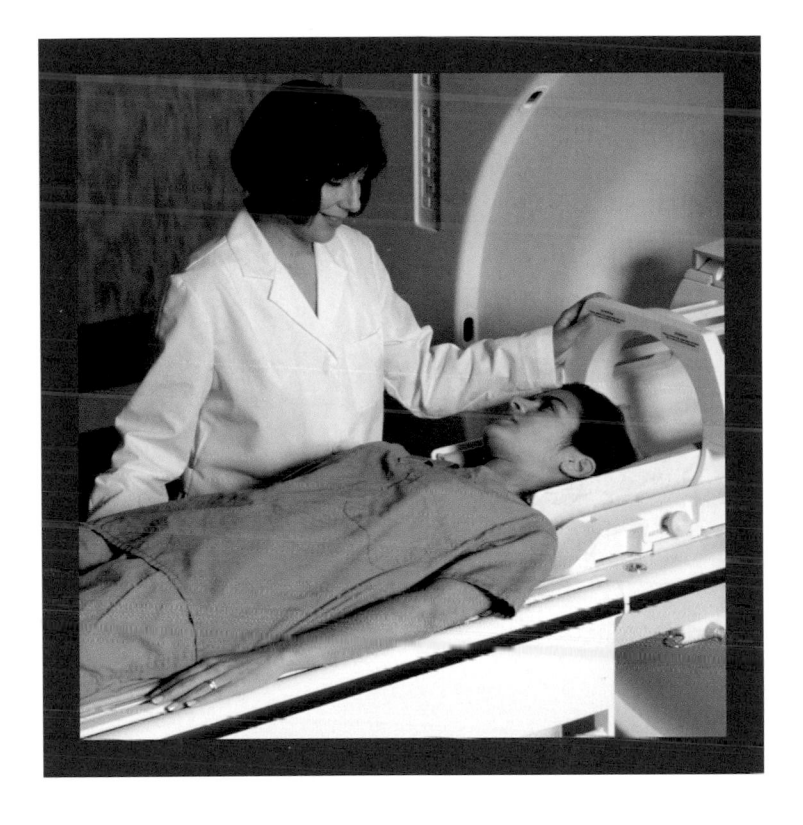

DEPRESSANTS ARE SOMETIMES USED TO HELP CALM PATIENTS PRIOR TO MEDICAL TESTS.

beliefs that the drug is necessary, or both. When used too often or in too great a dose, and especially when they are taken at the same time as other depressant drugs, they can become killers. They depress the activities of the CNS so much that basic functions, like breathing and heartbeat, become too slow or weak to keep a person alive. That makes depressants a common drug of choice for suicide. A survey of hospitals in 2002 found that about 45,000 people had been admitted to emergency rooms across the U.S. that year because of attempted suicide using benzodiazepines,

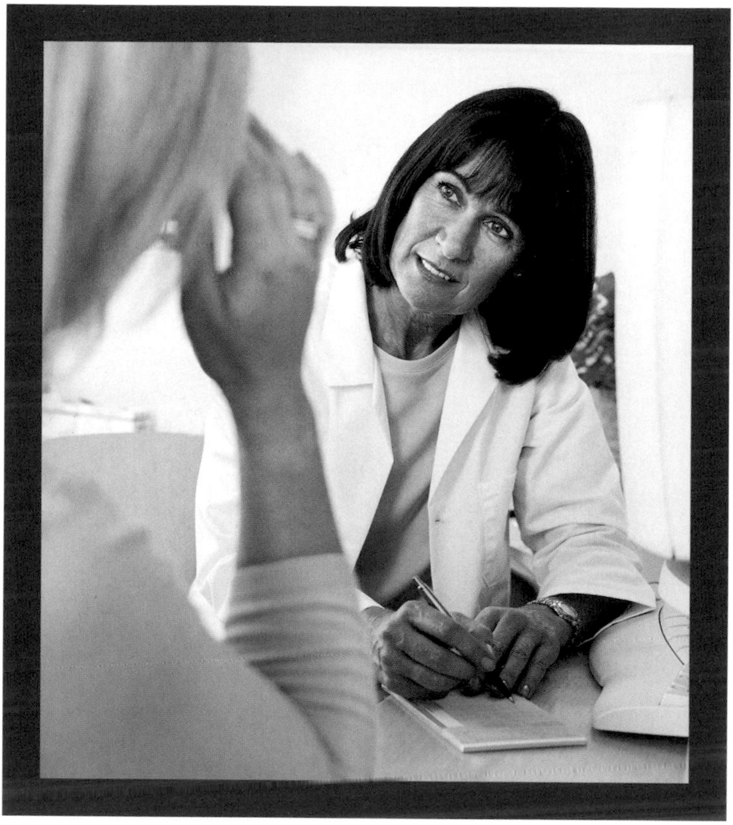

DEPRESSANT MEDICATIONS ARE LEGAL ONLY WHEN PRESCRIBED BY A DOCTOR.

the most common prescription depressant drug.

There are certain depressant substances that do not require a prescription. Alcohol is by far the most common. Because alcohol influences the brain and is not a natural component of the body, it is rightly considered a drug. And though there are laws against selling alcohol to minors, every high school student knows there are ways to get around the restrictions. Alcohol is not a primary focus of this book, which instead deals mostly with prescription and illegal depressants. But it will come into the discussion here because of its widespread use and the proven danger it poses when taken with prescription depressants.

There are also some substances in over-the-counter medicines that act like depressants. *Over-the-counter* means that anyone can buy them off the shelf from drugstores, supermarkets, or convenience stores. Some of the medicines that contain depressants are cold and cough remedies (which contain alcohol) and certain allergy medicines (which contain antihistamines). People who take these products usually are not doing so because of the depressant drugs in them, but because they contain other drugs that help relieve symptoms of temporary ailments.

Depressants are also available through several illegal routes. People who are addicted to a drug or want to try it as a "recreational" drug will steal it from other people: friends and family with prescriptions, doctors, dentists, veterinarians, pharmacists—anyone who might have a supply. The Internet has become a vast new marketplace for the illegal drug trade. Buying on the streets, at parties, clubs, and even at school are other common avenues. Drugs that have been made illegal in this country, like GHB (gamma hydroxybutyrate) and Rohypnol, can be purchased outside the country and smuggled across the border or sold on the Internet.

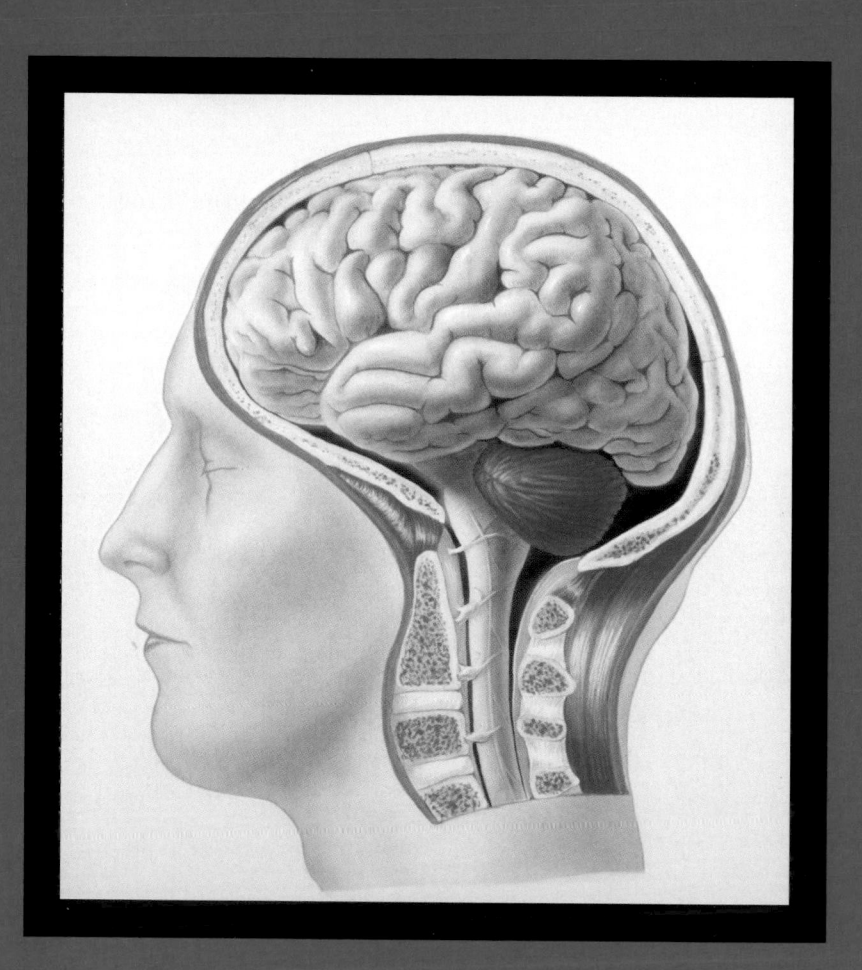

THE BRAIN AND SPINAL CORD MAKE UP THE CENTRAL NERVOUS SYSTEM, OR CNS.

2 HOW DEPRESSANTS INFLUENCE THE BRAIN

FOR CENTURIES SCIENTISTS have known that the brain is essential for keeping a person alive, as well as for such life-enriching things as laughing at a friend's joke, enjoying the flavor of a strawberry, feeling a desire to help someone in need, or learning to play a musical instrument like a virtuoso. But there is nothing about the appearance of the brain— a light pink, soft, bumpy orb—that gives any clue about how it does all that. The mystery began to unfold thanks to a remarkably simple yet powerful invention in the mid-1600s, the compound micro-scope. The microscope allowed scientists to discov-er that the brain and spinal cord were composed of cells now called neurons, plus other kinds of cells and many blood vessels.

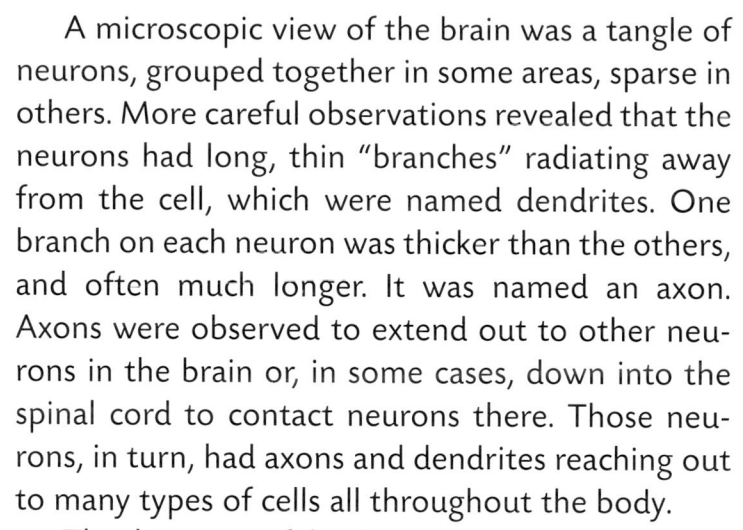

A microscopic view of the brain was a tangle of neurons, grouped together in some areas, sparse in others. More careful observations revealed that the neurons had long, thin "branches" radiating away from the cell, which were named dendrites. One branch on each neuron was thicker than the others, and often much longer. It was named an axon. Axons were observed to extend out to other neurons in the brain or, in some cases, down into the spinal cord to contact neurons there. Those neurons, in turn, had axons and dendrites reaching out to many types of cells all throughout the body.

The discovery of dendrites and axons, plus some experiments and logic, led scientists to recognize that communication was going on among the neurons. Dendrites receive information from other cells, while the axon sends information out. It became clear that the brain was part of a network of interconnected neurons that interacted with all parts of the body. It made sense that the brain, which contained a huge number of neurons, was the control center of it all.

But no one understood just how neurons of the brain and spinal cord worked together as a team until researchers began to explore the mysteries of what was going on inside neurons and at their surfaces. Such findings were made possible by new equipment invented in the last few decades of the twentieth century that allowed the tiniest amounts of substances to be extracted from neurons, identified, and measured. Clever reasoning and careful, tireless studies of brains from animals laid the foundation for today's understanding—though still incomplete—of just how the brain works and how drugs influence its activities. Cooperation among scientists helped, too, so that discoveries made in one laboratory could aid researchers in other laboratories in advancing their own studies.

Chemicals for Communication

Neurons are in constant communication with each other by means of chemicals called neurotransmitters. Neurotransmitters are like messages handed from one cell to the next. They are released by the tips of axons and become attached to the surfaces of adjacent neurons at special locations on their dendrites, or on the surfaces of the neurons. Virtually all drugs interfere in some way with the brain's neurotransmitter messages.

Using a comparison to students in a classroom to illustrate how the CNS works, a neurotransmitter message being passed between two neurons is like one student passing a note to a friend. The message is held out by the first student (like the neurotransmitter released by an axon) and placed in the hand of the friend (the neurotransmitter attaching to the second neuron's surface). An important detail is that the neurotransmitter attaches to a very specific area on the receiving cell, called a receptor. This would be like saying the note being passed must go

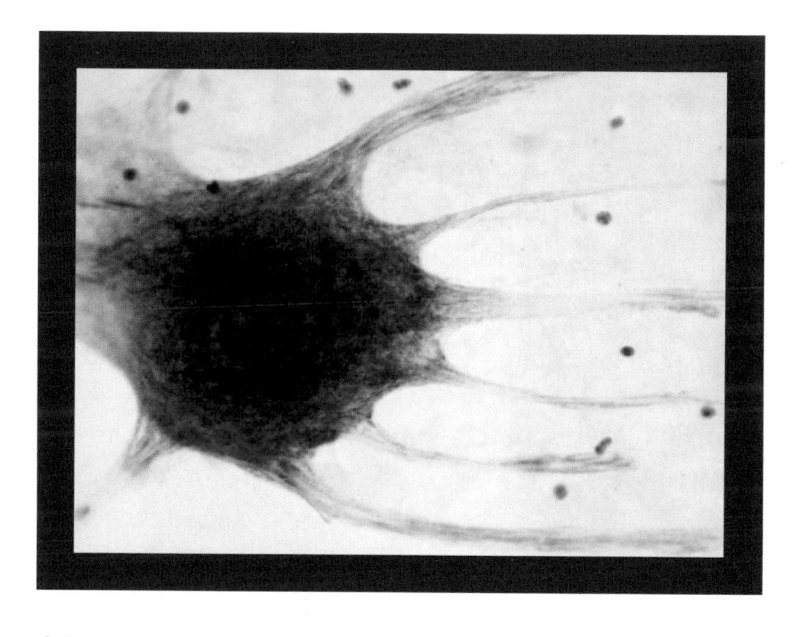

A NERVE CELL, OR NEURON. THE DENDRITES ARE SHOWN EXTENDING FROM THE CELL BODY. THE HUMAN BRAIN HAS ABOUT A HUNDRED BILLION NEURONS.

into the hand of the friend, not dropped on the floor, or put into a pocket.

What happens when the neuron receives a message? The neurotransmitter has attached to receptors, but then what? That depends on what type of neuron it is, and on the kind of neurotransmitter it is. In many cases, the receiving neuron is stimulated to carry out a task. Very often, that task is simply to pass the message along to another cell. Here's an example: if a person wants to get out of a chair, there are a group of neurons somewhere in the brain that have come up with this thought. They release the neurotransmitter from their axons, which attaches to receptors on other neurons in a nearby part of the brain. The message is "pass this along!" So those neurons, in turn, release a neurotransmitter of their own, which attaches to yet other neurons in the brain. Eventually, some of the neurons that receive the message are ones with long axons that leave the brain and interact with neurons in the spinal cord. Spinal cord neurons finally carry the message out to muscles that can move the legs and help get the person up. The message carried by those last neurons is "move!" In response, muscles contract and the person's body stands up as planned. (This last message, between neurons and muscle cells, also relies on neurotransmitters.)

The preceding example describes how neurotransmitters make something happen. Neurotransmitters that cause a cell to do something are called stimulatory neurotransmitters. But some neurotransmitters actually prevent cells from carrying out a task. Those are called inhibitory neurotransmitters, or simply, inhibitors. Their message to another cell is "don't do whatever other neurotransmitters are telling you to do."

Many different kinds of neurotransmitters—both stimulatory and inhibitory—are being released all the time within the brain (and spinal cord). Some scientists estimate that there may be hundreds of different neurotransmitters at work in the brain. Perhaps this makes sense, given all the different things going on in a brain, but

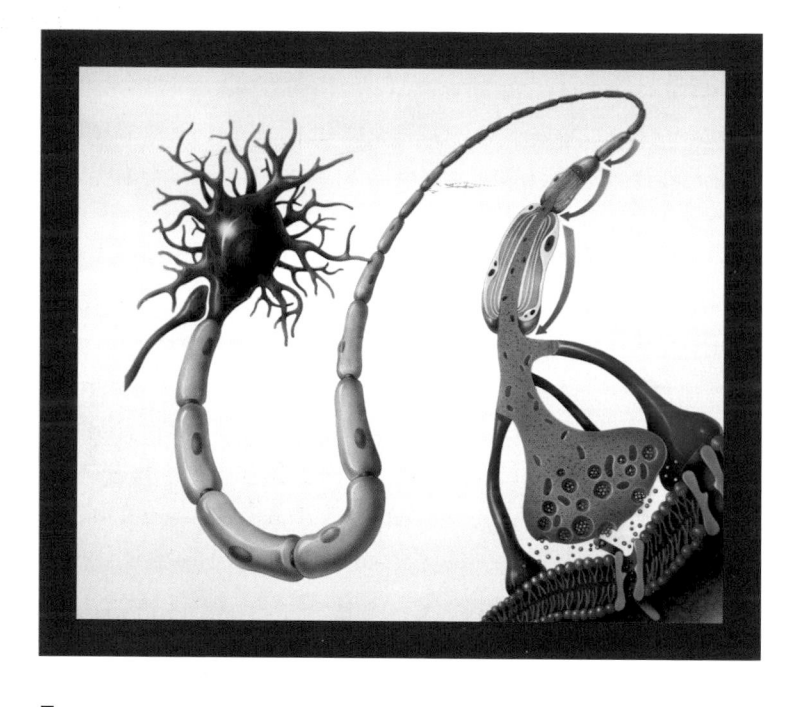

THIS ILLUSTRATION SHOWS A NEURON, AXON EXTENDED, RELEASING NEURO-
TRANSMITTERS ACROSS THE SYNAPSE TO THE RECEPTOR ON ANOTHER CELL.

it took scientists by surprise. Could it really be that complex? Yes. It is far more complex than that, in fact, as researchers continue to uncover amazing details about communication in the CNS. Some of the first neurotransmitters to be discovered are now well studied, but others have only recently been identified and little is known about them.

To summarize, neurotransmitters are chemicals that act as messages among the vast network of neurons in the CNS. There are hundreds of neuro-transmitters, which allow the brain to carry out an amazing number of different tasks. Some neuro-transmitters stimulate cells to do a task, while others inhibit cells from doing that same task. And it appears that a given cell is constantly getting lots of messages at once from many different neurons. If most of them say "don't," then the neuron will remain inactive, waiting for enough "do" messages to trigger it into taking action.

How Depressants Work

Virtually all depressant drugs interfere with a particular brain neurotransmitter called gamma-aminobutyric acid, or GABA. This extremely important brain chemical carries messages between neurons that control many of the body's activities, such as muscle control, breathing, sleeping, thoughts, memories, emotions, reasoning, and more. It is an inhibitory neurotransmitter.

Having a neurotransmitter like GABA may seem odd. However, this is just one example of the many ways in which the human body is controlled by a balance of opposing actions. It allows for faster, more accurate changes. It's like driving a car: having a brake and a gas pedal allows more control over the speed of the car than if there were only a gas pedal. Without a brake pedal, stopping would only happen by letting up on the gas, and it would take a while for the car to come to a full halt.

A healthy person has a balance between GABA and stimulatory neurotransmitters, which changes as needed. While a person is awake and active, GABA is helping to fine-tune the strength of messages being passed around the brain. But at some point GABA is released in greater amounts. This slows down brain activities, including its control of breathing, heart rate, and reflexes. Thoughts also change as certain neurons are inhibited from participating in the brain's communications. Eventually the person will feel drowsy and fall asleep. This is the body's way of shutting down some of its energy usage for a while, making time for repairing and rebuilding tissues.

GABA is also important in keeping the brain from becoming overstimulated while a person is awake. For example, a person can become very worried and anxious simply by thinking about certain things, like talking in front of the class at school. Some people are so concerned about saying something wrong or embarrassing, or are just so shy, that they literally feel sick. Neurons in their brain are frantically releasing neurotransmitters among neurons that are replaying thoughts like, "I can't do this," or "I'm going to do a horrible job!" Some neurons creating that thought pattern send messages to other areas of the body, causing physical reactions like sweating, trembling, chills, nausea, a pounding heart, and a dry mouth. These are all due to stimulatory signals racing around in the brain, triggered by fear, and passing along to the rest of the body. A person in this fearful state can learn to feel calmer by intentionally replacing thoughts of failing with images of doing a good job,

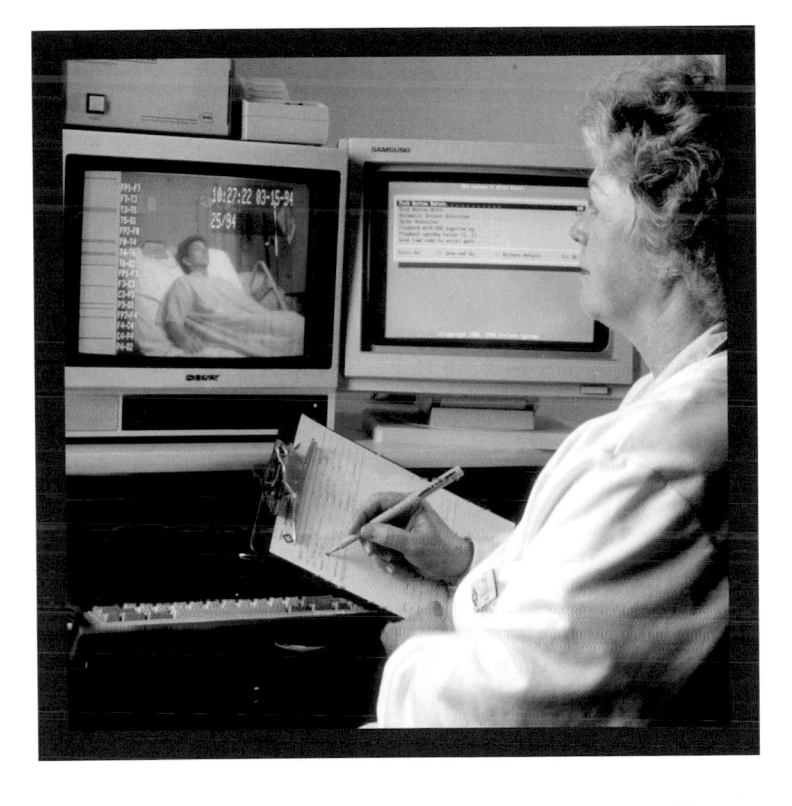

A RESEARCHER OBSERVES A WOMAN DURING A TEST ON SLEEP DISORDERS. GAMMA-AMINOBUTYRIC ACID, OR **GABA,** IS THE BRAIN CHEMICAL THAT CONTROLS SLEEPING, BREATHING, AND MUSCLE CONTROL. MOST DEPRESSANT DRUGS AFFECT **GABA.**

or by directing the presentation to a friend in the room as though it were a two-person chat. Doing so may cause neurons to release additional GABA, helping to balance out the stimulatory messages and reduce the physical signs of fear.

Virtually all depressant drugs exert their effects on a person by attaching to receptors for GABA. That somehow makes it easier for GABA to attach to neurons or to stay on longer once it already has attached. As a result, GABA's inhibitory effects are stronger than without the drug. That, in turn, pushes the neurons' balance toward an inhibited, inactive state. (Note that a few depressants, like ketamine and certain antihistamines, act through different neurotransmitters.)

Because the brain carries out so many different activities, any drug that causes changes in brain chemicals can have many effects. This is certainly true of depressants. In general, they replace anxiety with a sense of calm that has been described by some as "dreamy." They replace alertness and hyperactivity with sleepiness. They lessen behavioral inhibition—the hesitancy a person might feel about doing or saying things because of fear about how others might judge them. The inhibitory effect of depressants on neurons that control muscles causes slurred speech because of slow mouth, lip, and tongue movements. Other muscles are inhibited, causing slow or uncoordinated movements, which is why people taking depressants must not drive a car, operate machinery, or do other things that require physical coordination and quick reflexes. Another effect of depressants is slowed breathing. There are special areas of the brain that are responsible for sending messages to the muscles in the chest that fill and empty the lungs, and the neurons carrying those messages are inhibited by GABA.

The depressant drugs that are used medically have effects similar to those of alcohol, which is also a depressant substance. Someone can be "under the influence" of a prescription depressant, just as for alcohol. Similarly, someone who has taken an overdose of such a drug is said to be intoxicated, literally meaning to be suffering from its toxic effects.

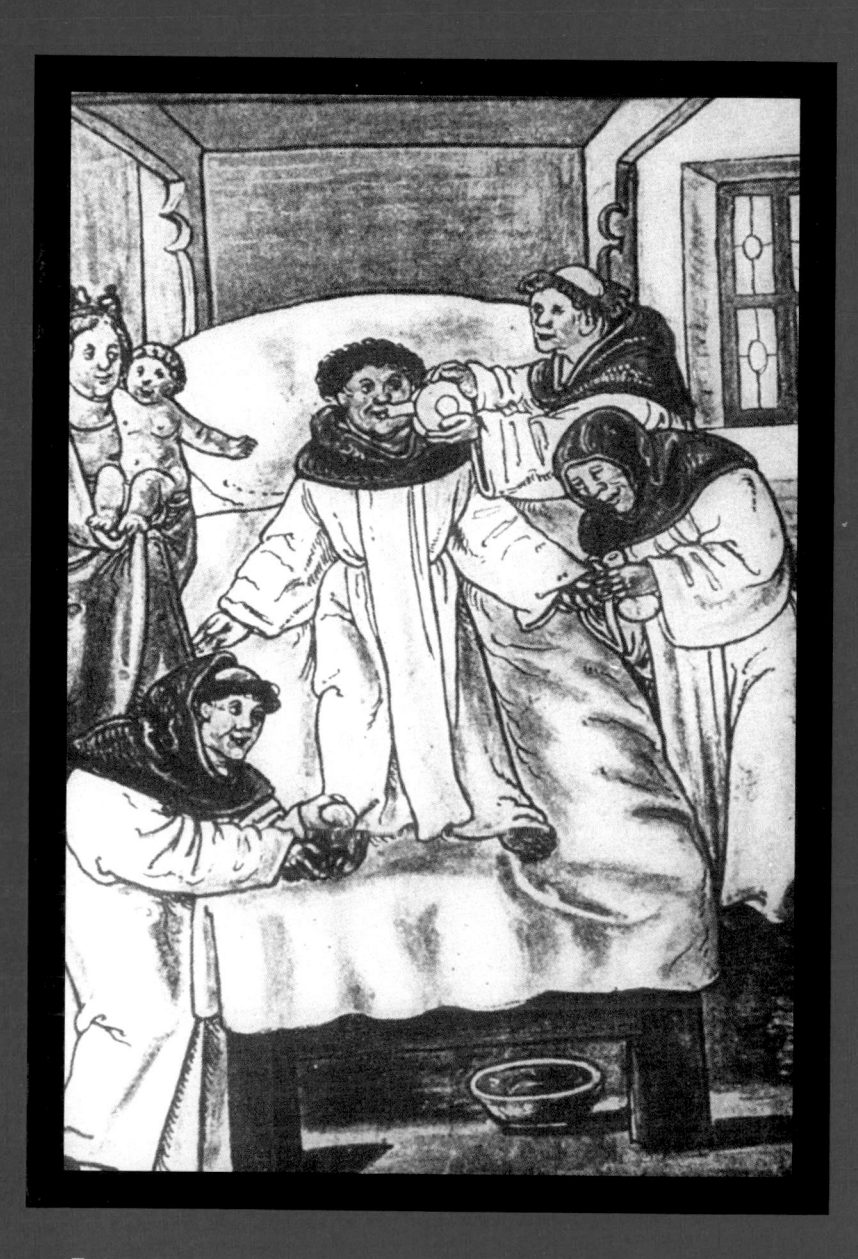

THIS ILLUSTRATION DEPICTS MONKS USING ALCOHOL AS AN ANESTHETIC.

3 A WHO'S WHO OF DEPRESSANT DRUGS

HUMAN SOCIETIES HAVE used plant substances for centuries to alter the way the brain functions. Some of those substances were sleeping aids; others helped a person relax during times of stress or reduced the agony of a painful injury. Some of those same plant materials are available today at natural-food stores or in the natural-food section of large grocery stores. Examples are valerian (a flowering plant) and kava (related to the black pepper plant), the roots of which are made into beverages for their sleep-inducing or calming effects.

Another plant substance that has been very popular for centuries for its CNS effects is opium. Opium is a thick syrup extracted from the outer covering of a particular species of poppy plant (*Papaver somniferum*). It causes relaxation and drowsiness when dried and smoked. Opium was once smoked quite openly, and still is in some parts of the world, although it is illegal in the United States. Its most widespread legal use now is in another form: the pain relievers morphine and codeine, extracted from the opium syrup. They are among the most valued plant products in medicine, but they are addictive. Other chemicals have been made from opium, including heroin, which have become major drugs of abuse. Dozens of other chemically related substances, all called opiates, have been created and are listed as controlled substances by the federal government.

Alcohol
One calming and sleep-inducing substance that people have turned to for all of recorded history is alcohol. Alcohol is produced in nature when plant materials are used as food by certain microorganisms that live in soil, by a process called fermentation. The effects of alcohol on the human body were discovered long ago, possibly when the earliest humans ate fermented grains or fruits. It dulls feelings, slows muscle control and coordination, causes sleepiness, and makes pain easier to bear.

Before there were prescription drugs for doctors to give to patients, alcohol was a common

01/23/12 01:14PM
Patron Name: STAUFFER, STEVE

The facts about depressants /
33020008011834   Date Due: 02/13/12

The science of addiction : from neurobio
33020500827430   Date Due: 02/13/12

Item Total: 2

Fines accrue at $ .20 a day per item

For renewal information, dial
303-404-5101

Renew your books by phone by dialing
303-404-5710
(Please have your library card ready.)

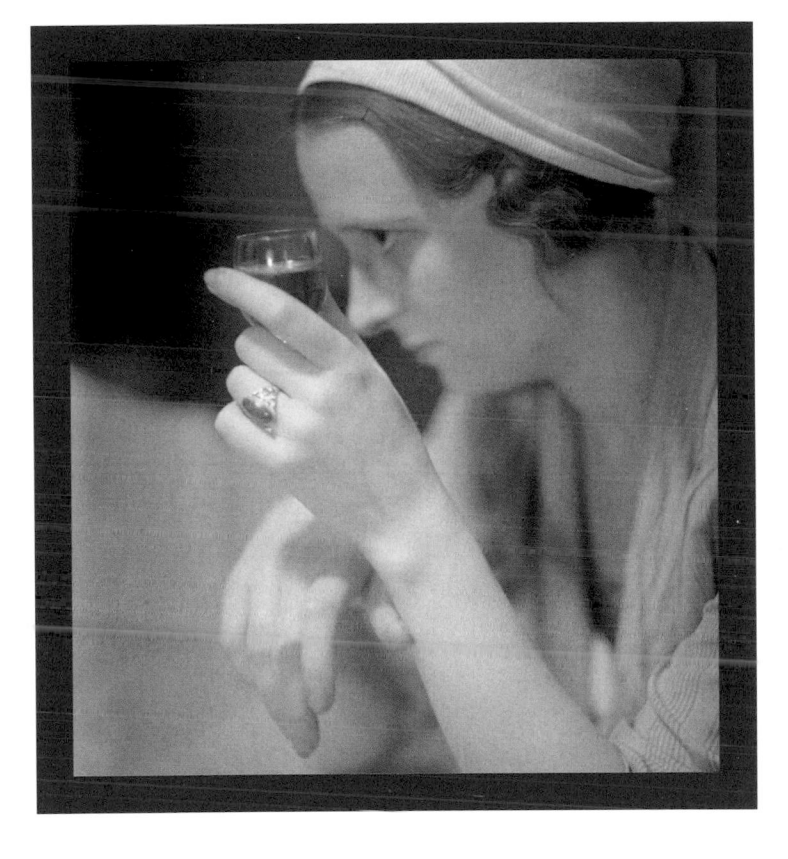

LONG BEFORE DOCTORS COULD PRESCRIBE DEPRESSANT DRUGS TO TREAT EMO-
TIONAL UPSET, PEOPLE TURNED TO ALCOHOL TO CALM THEIR NERVES.

remedy for people in emotional or physical distress. A gulp of strong alcohol often was the only thing a doctor could offer a patient needing surgery. It made the patient less aware of what was going on and less able to feel pain. Sometimes the alcohol would render the patient unconscious—a welcome state if the surgery had to be done without any other painkiller!

Even now, alcohol is included in a surprising number of over-the-counter medicines, especially treatments for colds and coughs. Some cough syrups contain as much as 25 percent alcohol, with the highest amount in those intended for nighttime relief of cold symptoms. Even children's cough syrups contain some alcohol, presumably to ensure the child will have a better night's sleep.

Today, alcohol is the most widely used depressant substance. Some people, especially if they are nervous, self-conscious, or shy, like the calming effect it produces. Even people who are comfortable among others enjoy "loosening up" with alcohol in social settings. But while social drinking may improve a person's feelings of enjoyment, the effects of alcohol can go far beyond that and include clumsiness, behavior changes, poor judgment, slurred speech, and other things that can be very unpleasant to witness or experience. Probably every adult, and some children and teenagers as well, can tell a story of someone who drank too much alcohol and who became loud, annoying, angry, or dangerous.

Barbiturates

The first group of drugs created specifically as sedatives can be traced back to 1863, when Adolph von Bayer (of Bayer aspirin fame) made a new compound in the laboratory of his chemical company. He called it barbituric acid, a combination of the

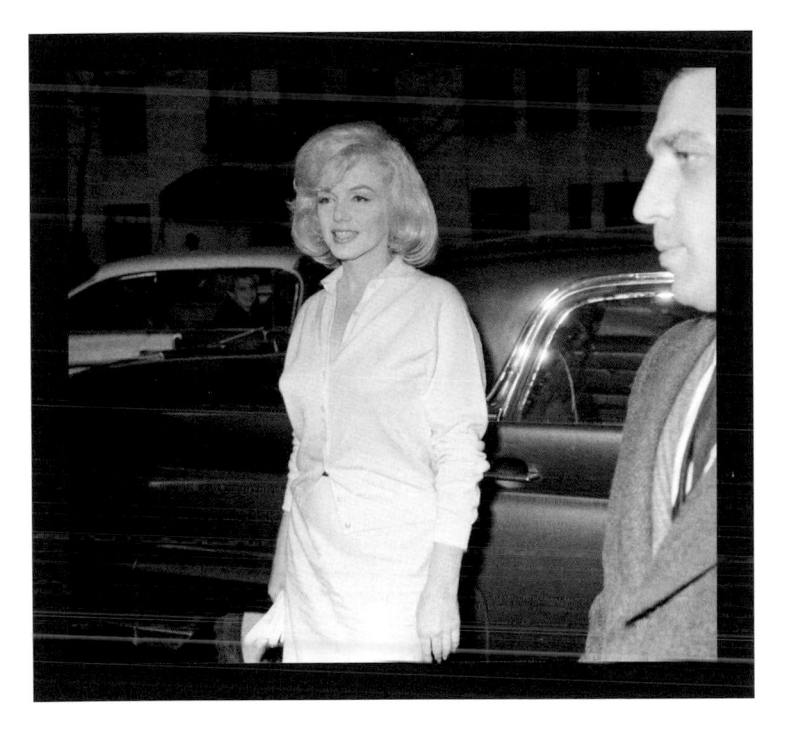

ACTRESS MARILYN MONROE LEAVING A NEW YORK HOSPITAL. IN THE SIXTIES, MANY PSYCHIATRISTS, INCLUDING MONROE'S, RELIED HEAVILY ON DRUG THERAPY. THIS APPROACH OFTEN LED TO DRUG DEPENDENCE. MONROE DIED IN 1962, AT AGE THIRTY-SIX, FROM AN OVERDOSE OF BARBITURATES.

type of chemical it was (a urate) and the special date on which it happened to be discovered: the feast day of Saint Barbara. That compound did not have any effect on the brain, but it was the starting material for a different chemical, barbitone, created forty years later in 1903. Barbitone, more often called barbital, was a colorless or white crystalline powder that turned out to be a strong CNS depressant. It became the first synthetic (artificial) sedative and was hugely popular as the earliest "sleeping pill."

In the years that followed, other drugs were created from barbital by changing small portions of the molecule. Over 2,500 different barbital-type molecules were eventually created in drug-manufacturing laboratories. Several were tested for their safety and effectiveness, first in animals, then in people. Today, a small group is still in use. They constitute the family of drugs known as the barbiturates. Many of their chemical names end with *barbital*.

The different kinds of barbiturates were found to have somewhat different effects. For example, some tended to make a person sleepy, while others created a sense of calm when upsetting events or anxious thoughts seemed overwhelming. Some barbiturates were even found to reduce seizures (convulsions) in people with epilepsy.

In addition to their medical uses, barbiturates soon became equally appealing to people looking for drugs to escape reality. In the mid-1900s, the problem of nonmedical barbiturate use began to surface as a national concern. They became known as thrill pills, taken for the altered perception they offered. But they also were known to be destructive to a person's life, because barbiturates are highly addictive and a few pills taken with a moderate amount of alcohol can be deadly. This combination of pills and alcohol sometimes happened accidentally, as when someone wanting relief from difficult emotional problems would have a few alcoholic drinks, then swallow a few sleeping pills to get some rest, not even realizing that he or she had taken too many.

Though the dangers of barbiturates became more apparent over time, their popularity continued until the federal government took steps to clamp down on their availability. In 1938 Congress passed the Federal Food, Drug, and Cosmetic Act, which put some restrictions on how medicines could be used. But it was the additional set of rules added in 1951, in what was called the Durham-Humphrey Amendment, that defined for the first time what kinds of drugs would be available only by a doctor's prescription. Any drugs that were known to be habit-forming qualified, and that included the barbiturates.

Although barbiturates fell behind in popularity after that, they are still used today as anesthetics and to treat epilepsy. Some are used by veterinarians to sedate or anesthetize animals for surgery. Barbiturates also remain active participants in the illegal drug scene.

Other depressant chemicals were created in an attempt to come up with something safer. Among them were meprobamate (sold as Miltown), glutethimide (Doriden), chloral hydrate (Somnos, Noctec), ethchlorvynol (Placidyl), and methaqualone (Quaalude, Sopor, Parest). None of these had major advantages over barbiturates, however. And though some are still in use today, most have been replaced in many physician's lists by the benzodiazepines.

Benzodiazepines

The most common depressants in use today belong to a group of drugs known as benzodiazepines. The first one, chlordiazepoxide (Librium), became available in 1960. It was soon followed by diazepam (Valium) and several others that were created by making slight changes in the basic benzodiazepine molecule. Today, benzodiazepines have replaced barbiturates as prescription sedatives and antianxiety medicines. One report concluded that a hundred mil-

Benzodiazepines used in the U.S.

GENERIC NAME	BRAND NAME	WHY IT IS PRESCRIBED
Alprazolam	Xanax	Anxiety plus insomnia
Chlordiazepoxide	Librium	Anxiety plus insomnia
Clonazepam	Klonopin	Anxiety, preventing seizures
Clorazepate	Tranxene	Anxiety plus insomnia; preventing seizures
Diazepam	Valium	Anxiety plus insomnia; preventing seizures
Estazolam	ProSom	Insomnia
Flunitrazepam	Rohypnol	Illegal use only; date-rape drug
Flurazepam	Dalmane	Insomnia
Halazepam	Paxipama	Anxiety plus insomnia
Lorazepam	Ativan	Anxiety plus insomnia
Midazolam	Versed	As a sedative in the hospital and before surgery
Oxazepam	Serax	Anxiety plus insomnia
Prazepam	Centrax	Anxiety plus insomnia
Quazepam	Doral	Insomnia
Quazepam	Doral	Anxiety plus insomnia
Temazepam	Restoril	Insomnia
Triazolam	Halcion	Insomnia

lion prescriptions for them were filled in 1999 alone.

Some benzodiazepines are short acting, meaning that their effects last for a few hours (though some people report feeling groggy or uncoordinated for many hours into the next day after taking a dose at night). These are mostly used for people who have insomnia—trouble falling asleep or staying asleep. Longer-acting types of benzodiazepines are prescribed for people who not only have trouble sleeping, but also have anxiety problems during their waking hours. Benzodiazepines are used in hospitals to sedate people with severe injuries or illnesses, or to calm patients awaiting surgery.

Besides taking effect very quickly, benzodiazepines have a big advantage over barbiturates: they don't have as great a depressant effect on breathing and so rarely cause death due to overdose (unless combined with alcohol or other depressants). Another advantage is that doctors can use a specific drug (flumazenil) to rapidly counteract the effects of benzodiazepines on the brain. This becomes useful when a benzodiazepine is used as a sedative or an anesthetic during minor surgery, because the counteracting drug can be given to make the patient alert as soon as the procedure is over.

Benzodiazepines have been described by some doctors as nearly perfect drugs. Those that are used to treat anxiety disorders, like panic attacks, bring relief within minutes, without causing sleepiness.

Other benzodiazepines are very effective in helping a person fall asleep, although many people say the ensuing sleep doesn't feel "normal."

But benzodiazepines are far from perfect. It was once thought that they wouldn't lead to dependence as the barbiturates did, but they do. Doctors now have differing opinions about how likely it is that a patient who uses benzodiazepines as directed—for no more than a few weeks—will become dependent on them. Some prescribe them without hesitation, while others are making every attempt to warn the public about the dangers. The drugs all come with strong written warnings about dependence. They have a variety of side effects, as do other depressants, such as loss of muscle coordination, mental fogginess and confusion, and amnesia. These negative effects may be downplayed or not even mentioned when benzodiazepines are prescribed.

One particular benzodiazepine, flunitrazepam (Rohypnol), has jumped into the national spotlight because it is being used to sedate people prior to sexual assault. This so-called date-rape drug is no longer legally available in the U.S., but continues to be smuggled into the country and sold through the Internet.

Imidazopyridines

A newer but very widely prescribed depressant is zolpidem (Ambien). It belongs to a class of drugs called imidazopyridines, along with zaleplon (Sonata). These drugs influence GABA in the brain, as do the benzodiazepines. They are used to treat short-term sleeping problems and are meant to be taken for a week or ten days, but people will take them longer if a doctor advises it. Zolpidem only takes about fifteen minutes to make a person feel sleepy. People taking this drug say it is important to get into bed immediately, because they have found that if they don't, they sometimes fall asleep somewhere else—like the bathroom floor—and don't remember how that happened.

It was hoped that these drugs would not create dependence, as do the benzodiazepines. But they do, and they share with those drugs the warnings about causing physical and mental impairments, including memory loss. Dangerous overdose when combined with other depressants, including alcohol, is a risk. Ambien also can create a sense of euphoria, or "high," and some people report having vivid dreams. Hallucinations and delusions are possible as well.

Azapirones
Unique, newer types of antianxiety drugs are the azapirones—buspirone (BuSpar), gepirone, and ipsapirone. They work differently than benzodiazepines. Rather than influencing the neurotransmitter GABA, they increase the abundance of receptors for a different brain neurotransmitter, serotonin.

I Thought I Was Dying

Magazine and television ads that encourage people to buy sleeping pills give the impression that the drugs solve countless problems and cause none. But Cathy tells a different story. Like many other people, she started taking sleeping pills to get through a difficult time. Cathy's mother was dying—at home, slowly, over three years. For months Cathy and other family members cared for her mother around the clock. As stressed and exhausted as Cathy was, she found she couldn't sleep when she had the chance.

To try and sleep Cathy did everything short of taking a drug. "I did meditation, good nutrition, detox teas and herbs, cut out things that might make you sick or keep you up, like caffeine, sugar, and I didn't watch violent TV late at night." But it didn't work. A woman who had rarely used medications in her life, Cathy finally decided to get some medical help.

> Our family doctor quickly gave me a prescription, saying there was no danger. He really thought the pills were lifesavers. So I took them and took them, until I finally thought I didn't need pills any more. But I got terrible rebound insomnia when I tried to stop.

She was told to take another type of medication that supposedly did not cause the same problems. She was assured it wasn't addictive. "I should have known better," she says. She hated how it made her feel. "When you take it, it's like a blackout. You wake up the next morning with a hangover. Your sense of time is altered, you're dizzy." So she tried to stop taking it. That was the beginning of what became a nightmare of physical and psychological reactions to the drug, and attempts to get off it. At times Cathy felt she might not survive.

"There was a period of time where I was absolutely sure that I had some kind of demonic possession. I used to make my husband tuck my sheets in a certain way so the gremlins wouldn't bite my feet." She also felt uncontrollable rage, very unlike her normal personality, and panic attacks, which she hadn't had before taking depressants.

"Sometimes I thought I was dying." She even considered suicide. Cathy sought out six medical experts to help her quit. Finally, over a two-year period, she made tiny dose reductions in a way that got her free.

The problem is that nobody is training doctors how to help you get off these drugs. The only thing they say is that if you are going to get off the drug, do it with supervision. Then they just say reduce the pill by a half, then a quarter, and so on. It doesn't work.

The azapirones do not cause drowsiness like many other antianxiety medicines do, nor do they appear to cause dependence as easily. They are used for mild anxiety problems, not for severe cases or for panic disorders.

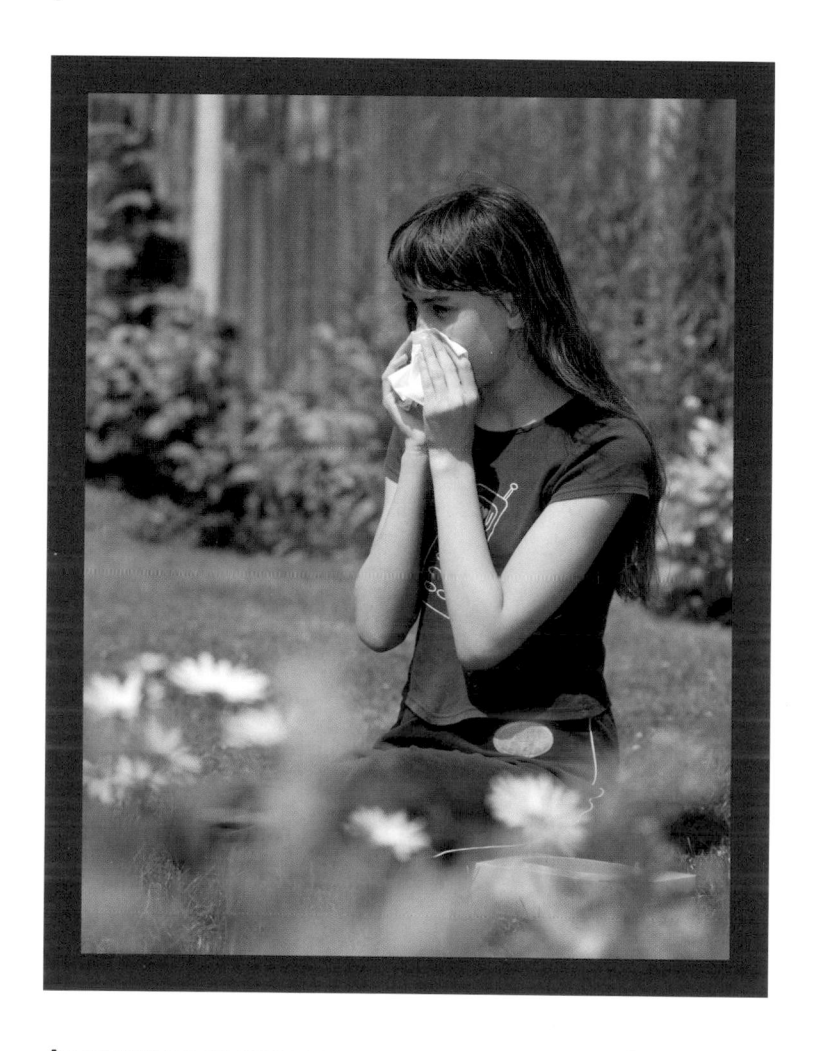

ANTIHISTAMINES ARE USED TO RELIEVE SYMPTOMS OF HAY FEVER. SOME OF THESE DRUGS HAVE SEDATIVE EFFECTS.

Antihistamines

Antihistamines are drugs that relieve symptoms of hay fever and other allergies. They are named for their ability to counter the effects of histamine, a naturally-occurring chemical that causes symptoms like a stuffy or runny nose, itchy eyes, and cough. Some of the antihistamines are different chemical beasts than the rest, and turn out to have some sedative effects on the CNS. They are sold in medicines that can be purchased at stores without a doctor's prescription because they are generally safe for most people.

One such antihistamine is diphenhydramine hydrochloride (trade name Benadryl). It is a very common ingredient in over-the-counter medicines. Another related drug is dimenhydrinate (Dramamine), which helps to prevent motion sickness. Both drugs influence one of the brain's very important neurotransmitters, acetylcholine. These drugs block acetylcholine's ability to attach to receptors, which causes drowsiness and some other typical depressant effects like poor coordination, irregular heartbeat, and short-term memory loss. Hydroxyzine (Atarax, Vistaril) is an antihistamine that is sometimes used to relieve anxiety and as a sedative, prior to medical or dental procedures.

High doses of these drugs are sometimes taken recreationally by people seeking an altered mental state. This abuse can cause hallucinations that are reported to be disturbing and unpleasant.

DO NOT DRINK ALCOHOLIC
BEVERAGES WHEN TAKING THIS
MEDICATION

TAKING MORE THAN RECOMMENDED
MAY CAUSE BREATHING
PROBLEMS.

MAY MAKE YOU DROWSY/DIZZY
THAT ALCOHOL MAY INTENSIFY.
USE CARE W/CAR-MACHINE

TAKING MORE ACETAMINOPHEN
THAN RECOMMENDED CAN CAUSE
SERIOUS LIVER PROBLEMS

THE FINE PRINT ON PRESCRIBED MEDICATIONS OFTEN WARNS AGAINST TAKING THEM BEFORE DRIVING OR OPERATING MACHINERY. MOST DEPRESSANTS AFFECT MUSCLE CONTROL AND ALERTNESS.

4 THE DOWNSIDE OF DOWNERS

ADVERTISEMENTS for hypnotics (sleeping pills) in magazines and on television show happy, fulfilled people enjoying their lives because they get a good night's rest using the advertised drug. But all depressants have side effects—undesirable alterations in a person's physical or mental state that happen as a result of taking the drug. These are the "fine print" warnings that accompany the bottle of pills or are listed on the back of magazine ads. Doctors and pharmacists are supposed to be sure patients understand the side effects of a drug before taking it.

A careful reading of the warnings will reveal quite a collection of possible side effects from taking depressants. Some are easy to handle, but others can be devastating. Some are rare, others common. Those described here are the most common, and they apply to virtually all of the different kinds of depressants being prescribed today. Some are short-term problems that happen while the drug is in the bloodstream. Others are long-term consequences of taking depressants for weeks, months, or longer.

Physical Effects

As the activity of the CNS is dampened by depressants, neurons that control muscle movements are less active. As a result, normal physical activities and reflexes can become slow and uncoordinated. A person under the influence of depressants, especially at higher doses, will have a difficult time walking properly and might stagger, trip, or even fall. Muscles that are used in talking are affected, causing slurred and slow speech. Some depressants cause muscle impairments more than others.

These changes in coordination and balance make it dangerous to drive a vehicle, use power tools, or do things that require physical skills, like playing contact sports, that could cause injury while under the influence of depressants and for several hours after their effects appear to have worn off. The time it takes to fully recover normal coordination after a single dose varies among people, and also depends on the specific kind of drug and quantity taken.

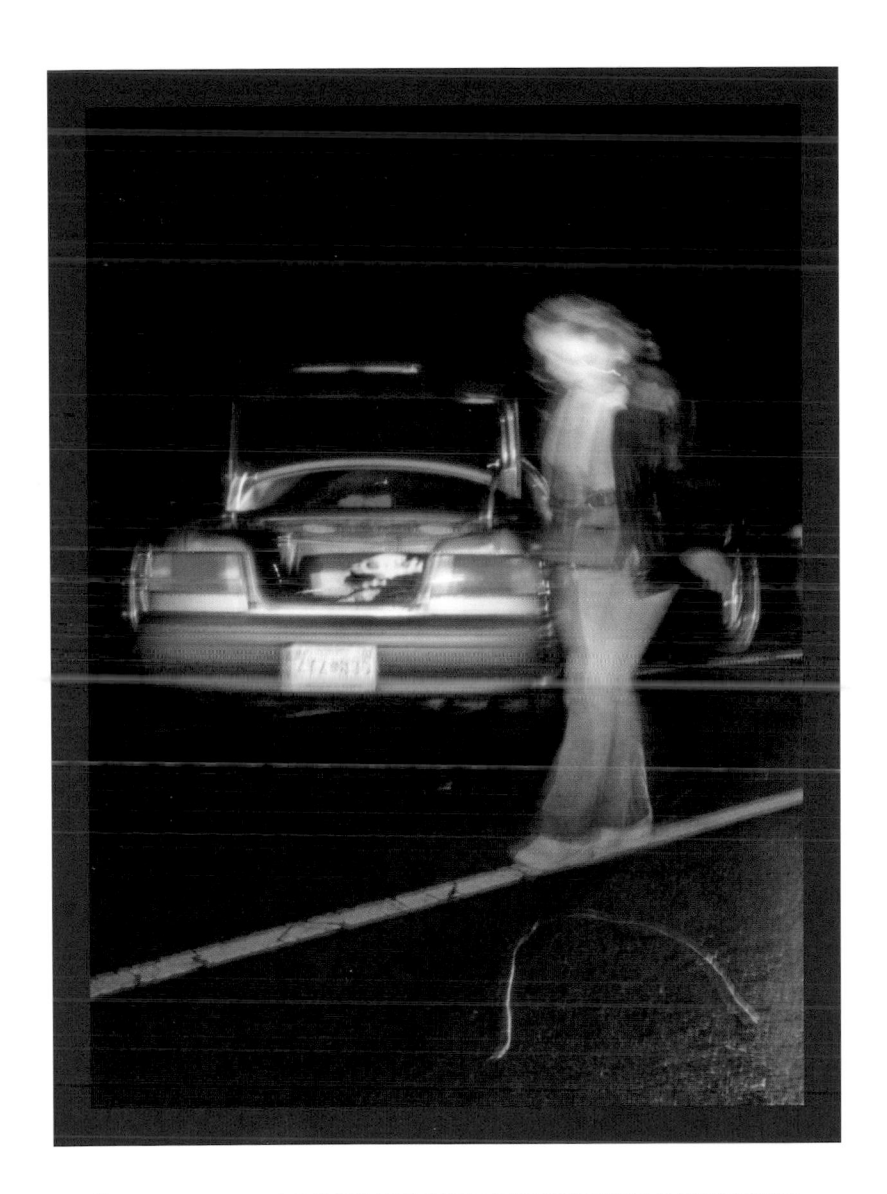

DRIVING UNDER THE INFLUENCE OF PRESCRIPTION DEPRESSANTS IS DISCOURAGED, BUT ONLY A FEW STATES HAVE LAWS AGAINST IT.

While it is illegal throughout the U.S. to drive under the influence of alcohol, only some states have laws that allow fines or imprisonment for people found driving under the influence of prescription depressants. Studies show that traffic accidents are more frequent among people who have prescriptions for benzodiazepines, especially during the first week of their use, than among people who are not taking them.

Mental Impairment and Memory Loss

Depressants influence the cognitive (thinking and perceiving) activities of the brain. They can cause muddled thinking, poor judgment, and difficulty in making decisions. An inability to form memories while under the influence is common. So someone who takes a sedative to help manage fear of airplane travel might be advised to takes a type of drug that wears off after just a few hours. Otherwise, if they are still under the influence while arriving at their destination, they may later have no recollection of how they got there. Memory impairment is also what makes date-rape drugs so insidious: victims who have been given a depressant without their knowledge often have little or no memory of whom they were with, which makes catching the perpetrator unlikely.

Depressants sometimes cause bizarre and disturbing thoughts, hallucinations, skin sensations, nightmares, and extreme emotional outbursts. And

Effects on the Adolescent Brain

Drug use by adolescents can have devastating long-term consequences. Recent research shows that major changes take place in the brain during adolescence. A process called "pruning" occurs in the brain at this time, in which some of the connections between brain cells are strengthened, while others are eliminated. Using substances that interfere with the developing brain can negatively affect processes such as memory and attention. Many scientists believe that this damage is irreversible.

while these appear to be temporary problems, evidence is accumulating that the use of benzodiazepines over several years may cause permanent changes in the brain. Studies show that certain areas of brain tissue are smaller than expected after long-term use—something called brain shrinkage. The data that shows this comes from studies in humans, not just in animals. But the number of people who have participated in such studies is still too small to decide how important an observation this is, but it is very disconcerting.

Emotional Blunting

People on antianxiety depressant drugs report that their emotions are not very strong—a problem called emotional blunting. This can seem a good thing if the person had been overwhelmed with anxiety, fear, or sadness—the drug is doing its intended job. But the feeling of pleasure is diminished as well. People describe feeling like a zombie, going through the day without much diversity in feelings, and having little interest in anything. That might be acceptable to someone whose anxiety had been devastating, but this blunting is a reason that some people stop taking depressants.

Tolerance
Regular use of depressants may lead to tolerance, which is the need to take more and more of a drug as time goes on to feel the same effect. For example, one antianxiety pill a day may relieve a person's distress for a few days, but over several days or weeks, the feelings of anxiety might not be controlled by just one pill. It will then take a greater amount of the drug to have the same antianxiety effect. Some people will take a higher dose, with or without medical advice, which perpetuates the problem. Sometimes a different depressant is prescribed, though tolerance can develop to the new drug as well.

Tolerance happens for a couple of reasons. One is that the neurons effected by the drug become accustomed to having it around and change because of it. Studies have shown that the GABA receptors, to which most depressants attach, become less abundant on neurons that are exposed to a depressant drug over time. With fewer receptors, there are fewer places for the GABA itself to attach, so

GABA's influence on neurons is lessened. Tolerance also happens because the body gets more efficient at inactivating and clearing the drug from the body. There are serious dangers related to tolerance. One is that if a person starts taking more of the drug to get the effect needed, that increases the body's dependence on the drug. It also pushes the person closer to a lethal overdose, because different parts of the brain become tolerant at different rates, and as more of the drug is taken for its desired effects, the parts of the brain that control breathing and heart rate don't become as tolerant. Instead, the life-giving activities of breathing and pumping blood are still sensitive to the lower dose of the drug and can become dangerously slowed as a person takes higher and higher doses.

Dependence
One of the strongest warnings against long-term use of depressant drugs is their ability to cause dependence—an overwhelming need to use a drug longer than originally intended, or after the reasons for which it was originally prescribed have been resolved. There are two types of dependence, both of which are at work with depressants. Physical dependence on a drug (also called addiction) is a change in the body's cells to a state where they require the drug to function. Psychological dependence is a belief that the drug is needed, whether the body has become physically dependent or not.

Recognizing Dependence

People are not usually eager to admit that they have a drug habit. It also isn't always easy to know if true dependence has developed. Some people who take a drug regularly, or who keep trying to stop only to start up again, swear that they aren't dependent. They say that they could stop any time if they wanted to, but they just don't want to. Recognizing dependence is the first step toward breaking the habit. Doctors have come up with a list of clues to help people determine whether or not they have a drug problem.

If the answer is "yes" to any of the three following questions, a person is considered dependent:

- Has the drug been taken for longer or in greater amounts than first intended?
- Is it proving impossible to stop taking it?
- Is a great deal of effort and time being put into getting the drug, or in recovery from its effects?
- Is taking the drug or attempting to get it replacing other activities like spending time with friends, family, at sports, at work, or in school?
- Does the user continue to take the drug even though it's clearly causing a physical or emotional problem, or making an existing problem worse?
- Is tolerance for the drug developing? Do symptoms of withdrawal show up when the drug is halted or its dose lowered?

Medications that are prescribed to people who need short-term help with sleeping are not meant to become a regular part of going to bed. They come with clear warnings that physical dependence can take hold if used for more than a few weeks. The same is true for barbiturates.

Most people for whom depressants are prescribed are trying to cope with a short-term problem. They benefit from taking the drugs for a brief time and then stop taking them without signs of dependence. But some people find it exceedingly difficult to stop because of severe withdrawal symptoms. These include intense anxiety and insomnia that lead individuals to assume they are still not well and must continue to rely on the drug they were taking. This dependence develops more often in people who take the depressant for longer than the recommended length of time.

In fact, there is a growing alarm about how many people in the country are within the grip of dependence to benzodiazepines. Doctor Edward Drummond is a physician and the author of *Benzo Blues*, a book that explains what many doctors aren't telling patients about how serious the problem of benzodiazepine dependence is. He and a few other doctors, plus several groups of past benzodiazepine users, are trying to alert citizens and the medical community that people need help getting off these drugs, and that they shouldn't be so readily prescribed in the first place.

Withdrawal

Withdrawal from depressants is one of their most serious dangers. The physical dependence that develops for prescription sleeping aids and antianxiety medicines develops so rapidly and is so powerful that patients are warned to consult a doctor before they stop taking them. When someone stops taking depressants, the brain's neurotransmitter balance is upset. Without the drug's inhibitory messages to which it had become accustomed, the brain can become overwhelmed with neurons' stimulatory messages—so much so that life-threatening seizures can be triggered.

The withdrawal reaction can include vomiting, abdominal cramps, uncontrollable trembling, excessive sweating, blurred vision, severe headaches, seizures, and more. In addition, emotional upheavals and distorted perceptions can be overwhelming. Sudden withdrawal can lead to extreme emotions, and even thoughts of suicide. Withdrawal frequently triggers "rebound" insomnia or anxiety that is far worse than before taking the drugs. People who experience the rebound assume their original problem is coming back and decide they must still take the drug, perpetuating their dependence. A feeling commonly described by people going through depressant withdrawal is that they feel like they are dying.

An alarming aspect of depressant drug withdrawal is that even a small reduction in dosage can trigger a severe withdrawal reaction. People are told to decrease their usage gradually when trying to get off these drugs, but neither they nor their doctors understand how tiny those changes in dose must be to avoid withdrawal altogether. What's more, many people are finding that it takes many months and even years to gradually come off these prescription drugs without experiencing extremely unpleasant symptoms in the process. Books, support groups, Web sites, chat rooms, and inpatient hospitals all are helping people to figure out how to get free of these drugs safely.

Overdose and Dangerous Mixtures

Lethal overdose, whether accidental or intentional, was one of the reasons that barbiturates were replaced by benzodiazepines as the drugs of choice for insomnia and anxiety disorders. For barbiturates, there is a fine line between the amount that works and the amount that can kill. Benzodiazepines are far safer, at least when taken alone, because their impact on breathing is less dramatic. However, people may end up taking dangerously high doses to compensate for tolerance. In addition, children can be poisoned or killed by an amount that wouldn't kill an adult.

As with overdose of one type of depressant, taking a combination of these drugs can cause insufficient breathing and heart function. This can lead to loss of consciousness, permanent brain damage due to oxygen deprivation, and even long-term coma or death. Prescription depressants should therefore never be taken while other depressant drugs or alcohol are in a person's system. It can be difficult to know if depressants are still lingering in the bloodstream because the effects of small amounts may not be obvious to the person taking them, especially if they have built up tolerance, and yet that amount could still pose a danger when other substances are added to the bloodstream. When in doubt, wait it out.

It is essential to remember that depressants also come in the form of prescription pain medicines that contain opiates (like morphine, codeine) and in some over-the-counter cold, flu, and allergy medications, which contain alcohol or depressant antihistamines.

Continued Anxiety or Insomnia

Another drawback of taking prescription depressants is that, for some people, drugs are a way to avoid healing the underlying problems causing the need for chemical help in the first place. Often there is a disturbing or painful incident in the person's past that created the problems. Post-traumatic stress syndrome is an obvious example of how this can happen, where being physically abused, for example, or witnessing abuse, leaves an imprint on the brain that continues to plague someone's life long afterward. Depressants can take the edge off those memories, and that is very helpful in the short term. Often the drugs alone do not bring mental stability. Use of these drugs in combination with therapy is considered the best way to reestablish a normal life without drugs.

Less traumatic reasons for taking sedatives or antianxiety medicines include sleeplessness and worry after losing a job, failing a year in college, going through a divorce, losing a friend or loved one, and other distressing events. And while drugs

The Sad Case of Karen Ann Quinlan

In 1975 a young woman from New Jersey became the first person whose "right to die" was fought out in a court battle between her family and doctors. At just twenty-one years old, Karen Ann Quinlan collapsed at a party. She had been drinking alcohol and also apparently took a Valium pill (a benzodiazepine sedative). The combination was too much for her central nervous system, and she collapsed, then went into a coma because the drugs depressed her breathing so much that her brain cells, without oxygen, were dying. She never came out of the coma and remained unresponsive to anyone or anything around her in a "vegetative state." Her heart continued pumping and blood flowed through her veins, but there was no sign that she was aware of anything going on around her. She gradually became emaciated (extremely thin), and lay curled in a fetal position. She sometimes blinked, grated her teeth, and even called out, but all were reflex actions.

Karen would not have survived long in that state if not for the life support machinery at the hospital that kept her breathing and receiving fluids and nutrients. Her family, after tests showed virtually no hope of recovery, asked doctors to remove the ventilator that kept her breathing. The doctors refused. After a famous court battle about Karen's "right to die," Karen's parents won and the breathing support was removed. To everyone's astonishment, she continued to breathe on her own. Sadly, she never came out of the coma. Karen Ann lived ten years in that condition, when she finally died of pneumonia in a nursing home.

Sleeping Better Without Drugs

One of the main reasons people take depressant drugs is to get a good night's sleep. But other things can improve nighttime sleeping and break the cycle of insomnia:

- Avoid caffeine, which is a CNS stimulant, especially in the evening. It is present in coffee, many teas, chocolate, cola drinks, and is added to some non-cola beverages like Mountain Dew.
- Create an environment in the bedroom that promotes sleep. This may mean getting a different mattress, pillow, sleepwear, or rearranging the room. Keep the room dark and quiet and minimize other sounds in the house as much as possible.
- Plan daily activities to enhance sleepiness in the evening, such as avoiding daytime naps, getting vigorous exercise during the day but not close to bedtime, taking a warm bath or shower before bed, avoiding large dinners or after-dinner snacks.
- Don't rely on alcohol—another depressant—to induce sleep! It may cause sleepiness at first, but can then cause middle-of-the-night wakefulness.
- Use slow, deep breathing or meditation techniques to relax the body fully when in bed. This helps to quiet stimulating thoughts and can induce sleep.
- Visit a doctor, naturopathic practitioner, chiropractor, or acupuncturist if physical discomfort might be part of the problem.
- Check with a natural food store, herbologist, or bookstore to learn which herbs can be used for their calming effects. (Warning: If you are taking a prescription or over-the-counter medicine, check with a doctor before also taking an herbal preparation. Some combinations can be dangerous.)
- Talk to a parent, friend, counselor, or therapist if there are feelings, thoughts, or situations that are causing anxiety.

can help, the anxiety or insomnia may actually be worsened or drawn out because of dependence on drugs. People aren't as likely to look for additional, longer-lasting help for their problems when their emotions are dampened by depressants. They may believe that drugs are the best help modern health care can provide anyway.

If tolerance develops, it seems like the symptoms are getting worse. In addition, a person who is distressed to begin with may next find himself or herself having to deal with drug dependence. What's worse, if a person tries to get off the drug and experiences rebound symptoms, that is often misinterpreted as proof that the drug is needed more than ever. This can keep a person enslaved to the idea of needing drugs to cope.

For all these reasons, turning to depressants for help is a mixed blessing. They can provide relief and hope to people with life-crippling psychological or emotional conditions. On the other hand, taking these drugs can also lead to a worse state of mental health, and adds the whole new threat of side effects. It is generally felt that the best way to use depressants is in combination with other healing strategies that make the drugs unnecessary as soon as possible. These include seeking help from a counselor or therapist as well as a doctor, getting practical help to recover from things like a lost job or career plan, finding a discussion group of people struggling with the same issues, and turning to friends and family who can be trusted and supportive even at the worst of times.

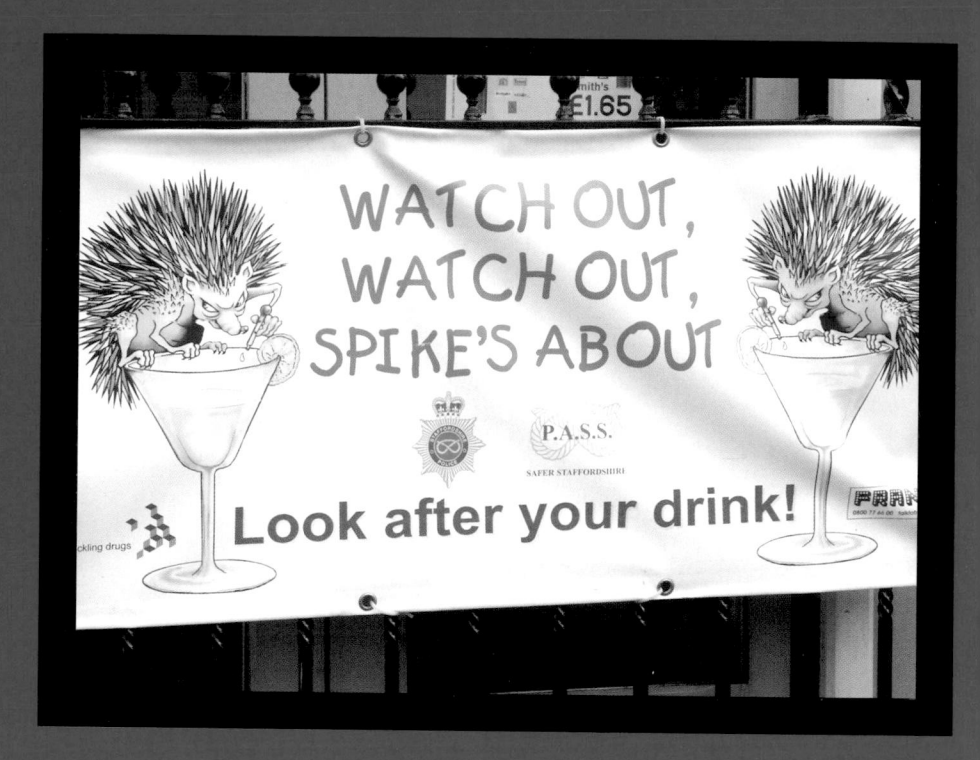

A SIGN OUTSIDE A BAR WARNS PATRONS TO KEEP AN EYE ON THEIR DRINKS. ROHYPNOL IS A TASTELESS AND ODORLESS DRUG THAT IS SOMETIMES SNUCK INTO DRINKS. WITHIN FIFTEEN TO TWENTY MINUTES, A PERSON CAN BE RENDERED UNCONSCIOUS AND MAY EXPERIENCE AMNESIA. SEXUAL PREDATORS USE ROHYPNOL IN DATE-RAPE CRIMES.

5 IN UNSAFE HANDS

THE CNS DEPRESSANTS have an important place among useful modern medicines. But they have become drugs of abuse as well. They circulate illegally and are used as mind- and body-altering substances for fun, with the unfortunate result of injuring or killing many young people. They also are being used as a weapon to sedate a victim who is then assaulted. The cat-and-mouse game of illegal supplies and users being sought by drug enforcement agents no doubt will continue for the foreseeable future. It is important that people educate themselves about the characteristics of drugs that are circulating and what the dangers are, both physically and legally.

Information presented here is likely to change over time as new laws are passed, new drugs become available, and methods of getting them shift. Readers are encouraged to stay on top of current events and to participate in drug education activities at school or in the community. It's the best way to make wise choices and stay safe.

Illegal Use of Depressants

Alcohol is the most widely available depressant in our society. It is legal now, though it hasn't always been. Today its sale and consumption have certain restrictions, such as the age at which someone can consume it. That restriction is meant to keep alcohol out of the hands of people who are believed to be too young to wisely choose when and where to use it, and how much. As is obvious from the hundreds of thousands of alcohol-related accidents, injuries, and deaths each year among people who are far older than the drinking age, the regulations do not prevent its abuse.

The other depressants, however, are controlled substances. That means it is illegal for anyone to buy, use, or possess them without permission from a doctor. (Exceptions are over-the-counter antihistamines, which are relatively weak in their effects, and drugs as they are handled by other medical workers and drug-making companies.) This is intended to keep depressants out of the hands of people who don't need them medically. And for those who do, doctors and pharmacists are supposed to ensure that the risks of taking the drugs are understood.

In addition, a doctor's prescription note tells the pharmacist exactly how many doses of the medicine a patient can buy at once. When those run out, a new prescription is needed. That prevents someone from having an excess supply of pills, which might be used for a suicide attempt, or could be sold or given away illegally to someone desperately looking for a supply without obtaining a doctor's permission. It also puts a limit on how long the drug can be taken, which reduces the chance of becoming dependent.

Of course, doctors can't control everything a person does. A controlled substance can still be acquired if someone really wants to get it. Depressant drugs are sought by some people for recreational use—for the altered feelings they cause. The depressants are not nearly as popular as drugs that give a sense of euphoria or a "rush" of energy. It is difficult to estimate how many people use them recreationally because of the millions of prescriptions that put them legally into household medicine cabinets, from which they are easily sampled. Users tend to be adolescents experimenting with drugs, and people in the club and party scene. In addition, people taking cocaine, which has a stimulating effect on the brain, report using depressants, or "downers," as they are called, to create just the balance of drug effects they want.

But how do people get hold of depressants, other than by sampling from someone else's prescribed allotment? One way is by giving false information about symptoms to a doctor. This can be repeated with other doctors, including those in other cities and states. Some people get their illicit drugs through person-to-person purchase. Buying drugs through the Internet is a another practice that is extremely difficult for law enforcement to control. And prescription drugs are sold in other countries, sometimes over the counter, and can be purchased while on a trip and carried across the border. Though rare, doctors sometimes participate in the misuse of drugs by writing prescriptions that are not necessary, but doctors' prescription records can be checked by drug control authorities to look for suspicious activities like excessive prescribing of certain drugs.

Controlled Substances and the Law
In 1970, the U.S. Congress decided that there should be regulations in place to control the availability and use of the many drugs—both medicinal and recreational—that were becoming available to the public. The Controlled Substances Act was created, and is still the basis for laws about drugs today.

The act determined that several types of drugs should be controlled. Those included depressants, as well as narcotics, stimulants, hallucinogens, anabolic steroids and the chemicals used to make such drugs. It became illegal to sell, manufacture, distribute, cultivate, or possess a "controlled" substance without proper authority. Each drug was then put into one of five categories, called schedules. The schedules ranked drugs by the risk of addiction or abuse and how important they were as medicines. Schedule I drugs were the most dangerous and of little or no medical use. Schedule V drugs had little likelihood of being abused and were useful in medical treatment. These schedules are still in use today, though a drug's position in the listing can be changed as information about it changes. A drug's ranking helps lawmakers to determine appropriate punishment for involvement with illicit drugs. In general, the lower the schedule number the more severe the punishment.

One depressant that is listed in Schedule I is methaqualone. In the 1960s and 1970s, this drug was present in sleeping aids Quaalude, Sopor, and Parest. As drugs of abuse, the pills were often called "ludes." In 1984 methaqualone was listed as a Schedule I substance when it became clear that it was as dangerous as barbiturates in causing tolerance and dependence. It is no longer legally produced in the U.S.

A far more troubling drug is gamma hydroxybutyrate (GHB). This Schedule I drug is illegal for doctors to prescribe, but it is still abundant on the illegal drug market. GHB has been reported to cause many emergency room visits, hospitalizations, and deaths. It is also used to sedate rape victims. Another date-rape drug, Rohypnol (a benzodiazepine), wasn't expected to become the notorious drug of abuse that it has. It recently joined GHB among the Schedule I substances. In 1996, Congress passed the Drug-Induced Rape Prevention and Punishment Act. This act increased the punishment to up to twenty years imprisonment for any person who distributes a controlled substance, like GHB or Rohypnol with the intention of making a person vulnerable to sexual assault or other violent crime.

Club Drugs
All-night dance parties, or raves, are places for teens

and young adults to enjoy music, dance, and social- ize. They have also been places where young people experiment with drugs. At some parties, drugs are a small, secret part of the activities. At others, the flow of illegal substances is widespread. In previous gen- erations, alcohol was the most common substance used illegally, and that is still true. But other CNS depressants are popular on the party and club scene. They are taken to experience the unusual feelings and thoughts they create, often very quickly. But they also are being used as weapons for criminal pur- poses—to sedate an unsuspecting person who then is assaulted or raped. These drugs, called "predatory drugs" when used this way, make a victim confused and too weak to fight back. In addition, they cause amnesia, so it is difficult for someone who has been abused to remember what happened and who did it.

The most common depressants on the club and party scene are GHB, Rohypnol, and ketamine They are colorless and can be slipped easily into drinks without a person's knowledge. Such small quanti- ties can be used that they don't change the flavor of the beverage. That is why people who attend par- ties are being strongly warned to keep track of their beverage at all times, to never leave it sitting around unattended, and never accept a beverage that someone else has poured or offers to share.

Knowing the effects of these drugs is important and might save a life, yet they can be difficult to tell apart from the effects of too much alcohol. But if someone has not had alcohol, or only a small

Common Names for Club Drugs

GHB (gamma hydroxybutyrate): Cherry Menth, Easy Lay, G, GBH, Gamma-OH, Georgia Home Boy, Goop, Grievous Bodily Harm, G-Riffick, Liquid E, Liquid Ecstasy, Liquid X, Organic Quaalude, Salty Water, Scoop, Soap, Vita-G

Rohypnol (flunitrazepam): Forget me pill, Mexican valium, Pingus, R-2, Reynolds, Rib, Roach, Roach-2, Roaches, Roapies, Robutal, Roofies, Rope, Rope marijuana, Rophies, Rophy, Ropies, Roples, Row-shay, Ruffies, Ruffles, The lunch money drug, Wolfies

Ketamine: Cat Valium, Green, Jet, K, Special K, Super Acid

amount, and is behaving as though drunk, with poor muscle coordination, slurred speech, excessive tiredness, dizziness, mental confusion, bizarre thoughts, emotional outbursts, or other unexpected behaviors, they may have been given (or taken voluntarily) one of these drugs.

Because death by respiratory depression is a real danger and has killed dozens of people, getting medical attention could mean the difference between life and death. Calling an ambulance is better than trying to drive a person to the hospital, because emergency medical personnel arrive quickly and bring emergency equipment and expertise with them.

Mexico and Canada and purchasing it on the Internet.

Two other drugs similar to Rohypnol are becoming more common as drugs of abuse in some parts of the U.S. These are clonazepam (Klonopin) and alprazolam (Xanax), both prescription benzodiazepines. They are legal, but like all benzodiazepines, require prescriptions if purchased in the states. The source for recreational use appears to be mostly from outside the borders, especially Mexico.

Ketamine

Ketamine comes as a clear liquid or white powder that is used as an anesthetic during surgery, both for people and for animals (hence, one of its nicknames, "cat valium"). It depresses the CNS in a manner different from that of benzodiazepines and barbiturates, without influencing the neurotransmitter GABA. Just how it works is not entirely clear, though it may interfere with more than one of the brain's other stimulatory neurotransmitter messaging systems.

Ketamine is a controlled substance available only to veterinarians and doctors. Abusers of the drug have stolen it from veterinary offices, as well as imported it from other countries. People who take it voluntarily do so for the altered perceptions it creates, which some have described as an out-of-body or near-death experience. It is added to drinks or smoked materials (tobacco, marijuana), or is injected or snorted. It is also slipped into drinks of intended victims of assault. At higher doses, ketamine can cause mental confusion, amnesia, high blood pressure, and severe breathing problems.

Is It Worth It?

People who use drugs illegally and are caught may get lucky and receive nothing worse than a warning or a fine. Or, they may be told to do some hours of community service, or have to spend time living in a detention center or rehabilitation center. Other possibilities are more grave, however, and can change someone's life forever. Punishments for illegal use, possession, or sale of controlled substances can include going to prison, paying huge sums of money in fines, court fees, and lawyer fees, and losing possessions like cars that can't be paid for while in prison. Being in prison means no income and nothing to support family members who may have relied on the person behind bars. Parents who are convicted of drug crimes might lose custody of their children.

Kids Keep Getting Smarter

Teenagers are more aware of the dangers associated with drug abuse than they were a decade ago. That is according to a 2004 survey of teen drug use conducted by the National Institute on Drug Abuse (NIDA), a U.S. government agency that collects information about drugs and their usage. The number of high school students using illegal drugs is the lowest it has been for a decade. According to the survey, the most commonly used drugs in 2003 were alcohol, marijuana, ecstasy, Vicodin, OxyContin, and tobacco. Students reported less usage of depressants in recent years.

Getting caught using drugs illegally can also ruin plans for a good career. An illegal drug user will probably lose any current job and will seriously hinder his or her chances of being hired in the future. Any employer has the right to ask, "Have you ever been arrested or convicted of a crime?" If the answer is "yes," the job interview is usually over.

People who use drugs to influence other people, like slipping GHB into somebody's drink, are committing a crime even more serious than taking illegal drugs themselves. To do so is violence against another person, an action that may even endanger that person's life. Combined with other actions like rape or assault, the sentence handed down in court for such crimes could be years in prison.

GLOSSARY

addiction: The condition of having a physical need for a substance. See also dependence.

barbiturates: A group of drugs made from the compound barbital (barbitone) and which are strong CNS depressants.

coma: A state of deep unconsciousness from which a person cannot be awakened.

controlled substance: A substance listed by the federal government as potentially dangerous for health or abuse reasons.

CNS: Central nervous system, consisting of the brain and spinal cord, which controls virtually every life-sustaining and life-enriching activity of the body.

delusion: An idea that something is real, even though it is not possible.

dependence: The physical or psychological need for something that causes a person to devote much time, attention, and/or money to obtaining that thing. Physical dependence on a drug (addiction) is a change in body chemistry that makes continued use necessary to avoid withdrawal symptoms. Psychological dependence is a powerful desire for the drug, but without physical symptoms of withdrawal if it isn't taken.

drug of abuse: A medicine or other substance used in a way other than to help with a medical problem, often with the risk of causing physical or mental harm.

euphoria: Feeling of extreme happiness or wonderment.

GHB: Gamma hydroxybutyrate, a very dangerous "club drug" that has been used to sedate victims for sexual crimes.

hallucination: An imaginary experience perceived by the senses, as in seeing and hearing things that are not present.

hypnotic: A substance that causes sleepiness.

insomnia: A condition of being unable to fall asleep, sleep deeply, or sleep long enough to be healthfully rested.

intoxication: An altered state of awareness or of physical condition due to a substance taken into the body, often with the risk of being harmful (toxic). (Not just alcohol, but drugs are spoken of as causing intoxication.)

lethal: Causing death.

neuron: A cell in the brain, spinal cord, or in other areas of the body involved in coordinating thoughts, feelings, sensations, movements, and more.

recreational drug: A substance taken for the effects it has on the brain and body as a kind of entertainment rather than for any medical need.

sedative: A substance that helps a person feel calm and sometimes, sleepy.

seizure: A short (a few seconds to minutes) period of abnormal brain activity that can cause uncontrolled muscle contractions in the body, or unusual sensations, behaviors, awareness, or thoughts. Some seizures cause such strong muscle contractions as to become life threatening. Also called a convulsion.

side effect: An effect that a drug (medicine) has on the body, other than the one(s) for which it is being taken.

tolerance: The condition in which a person's body becomes accustomed to a drug, so that, over time, its effects become weaker. Higher doses of the drug are then needed to have the same effect that a lower dose once had.

withdrawal: The process of discontinuing the use of a drug, which can cause severe physical, emotional, or mental changes.

FURTHER INFORMATION

Web Sites

www.deatip.net/—Teens in Prevention (TiP), a network of school-based community organizations of young people seeking to reduce substance abuse and violence.

www.teens.drugabuse.gov/—Real stories, facts, questions, and answers about drugs, especially designed for teenagers by the National Institute on Drug Abuse (a subdivision of the National Institutes of Health).

www.drugabuse.gov/NIDAHome.html—The National Institute on Drug Abuse's page for news about drug research, usage, and abuse, with links to many additional resources.

www.clubdrugs.org/—Information about club drugs and how to stay safe, sponsored by the National Institute on Drug Abuse.

www.usdoj.gov/dea/—News and information about drugs and the law, sponsored by the U.S. Department of Justice's Drug Enforcement Administration.

www.darksideofsleepingpills.com/ch2.html—An excellent, doctor-written e-Book online, *The Dark Side of Sleeping Pills* by Daniel F. Kripke, M.D.

Organizations to Contact

These organizations provide information regarding drug and alcohol use and can make referrals to local resources.

Al-Anon/Alateen
1600 Corporate Landing Parkway
Virginia Beach, VA 23454-5617
Phone: 888-4AL-ANON
www.al-anon.alateen.org/

National Clearinghouse for Alcohol and Drug Information (NCADI)
P.O. Box 2345
Rockville, MD 20847-2345
Phone: 800-729-6686
www.ncadi.samhsa.gov/

National Council on Alcoholism and Drug Dependence, Inc. (NCADD)
12 West 21 Street, 8th Floor
New York, NY 10010
Phone: 212-206-6770
www.ncadd.org/

National Drug Intelligence Center
319 Washington Street, 5th Floor
Johnstown, PA 15901
Phone: 814-532-4601
www.usdoj.gov/ndic/

BIBLIOGRAPHY

Breggin, Peter R., and David Cohen. *Your Drug May Be Your Problem: How and Why to Stop Taking Psychiatric Medications*. Reading, MA: Perseus Books, 1999.

Drummond, Edward H. *Benzo Blues: Overcoming Anxiety Without Tranquilizers*. New York: Plume Books, 1998.

Kuhn, Cynthia, et al. *Buzzed: The Straight Facts about the Most Used and Abused Drugs from Alcohol to Ecstasy*, 2nd Ed. New York: W.W. Norton & Company, 2003.

Thomson PDR. *The PDR Pocket Guide to Prescription Drugs*, 6th Ed. New York: Simon & Schuster Adult Publishing Group, 2003.

Trickett, Shirley. *Free Yourself from Tranquilizers and Sleeping Pills*. Berkeley, CA: Ulysses Press, 1997.

Weil, Andrew, and Winifred Rosen. *From Chocolate to Morphine: Everything You Need to Know About Mind-Altering Drugs*. Boston: Houghton Mifflin Co., 1998.

INDEX

ABOUT THE AUTHOR

Lorrie Klosterman, Ph.D., has been a writer and educator in the biological and medical sciences for two decades. She earned a doctorate from the University of California at Berkeley and continues to enjoy learning about the wonders of science every day.